Lecture Notes in Computational Vision and Biomechanics

Volume 17

For further volumes:
http://www.springer.com/series/8910

The research related to the analysis of living structures (Biomechanics) has been a source of recent research in several distinct areas of science, for example, Mathematics, Mechanical Engineering, Physics, Informatics, Medicine and Sport. However, for its successful achievement, numerous research topics should be considered, such as image processing and analysis, geometric and numerical modelling, biomechanics, experimental analysis, mechanobiology and enhanced visualization, and their application to real cases must be developed and more investigation is needed. Additionally, enhanced hardware solutions and less invasive devices are demanded.

On the other hand, Image Analysis (Computational Vision) is used for the extraction of high level information from static images or dynamic image sequences. Examples of applications involving image analysis can be the study of motion of structures from image sequences, shape reconstruction from images and medical diagnosis. As a multidisciplinary area, Computational Vision considers techniques and methods from other disciplines, such as Artificial Intelligence, Signal Processing, Mathematics, Physics and Informatics. Despite the many research projects in this area, more robust and efficient methods of Computational Imaging are still demanded in many application domains in Medicine, and their validation in real scenarios is matter of urgency.

These two important and predominant branches of Science are increasingly considered to be strongly connected and related. Hence, the main goal of the LNCV&B book series consists of the provision of a comprehensive forum for discussion on the current state-of-the-art in these fields by emphasizing their connection. The book series covers (but is not limited to):

- Applications of Computational Vision and Biomechanics
- Biometrics and Biomedical Pattern Analysis
- Cellular Imaging and Cellular Mechanics
- Clinical Biomechanics
- Computational Bioimaging and Visualization
- Computational Biology in Biomedical Imaging
- Development of Biomechanical Devices
- Device and Technique Development for Biomedical Imaging
- Digital Geometry Algorithms for Computational Vision and Visualization
- Experimental Biomechanics
- Gait & Posture Mechanics
- Multiscale Analysis in Biomechanics
- Neuromuscular Biomechanics
- Numerical Methods for Living Tissues
- Numerical Simulation
- Software Development on Computational Vision and Biomechanics
- Grid and High Performance Computing for Computational Vision and Biomechanics
- Image-based Geometric Modeling and Mesh Generation
- Image Processing and Analysis
- Image Processing and Visualization in Biofluids
- Image Understanding
- Material Models
- Mechanobiology
- Medical Image Analysis
- Molecular Mechanics
- Multi-Modal Image Systems
- Multiscale Biosensors in Biomedical Imaging
- Multiscale Devices and Biomems for Biomedical Imaging
- Musculoskeletal Biomechanics
- Sport Biomechanics
- Virtual Reality in Biomechanics
- Vision Systems

Jianhua Yao · Tobias Klinder
Shuo Li
Editors

Computational Methods and Clinical Applications for Spine Imaging

Proceedings of the Workshop held at the 16th
International Conference on Medical Image
Computing and Computer Assisted
Intervention, September 22–26, 2013,
Nagoya, Japan

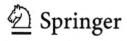 Springer

Editors
Jianhua Yao
Center Drive
National Institutes of Health
Bethesda, MA
USA

Shuo Li
GE Healthcare and University of Western
  Ontario
London, ON
Canada

Tobias Klinder
Innovative Technologies Research
  Laboratories
Philips Research
Hamburg
Germany

ISSN 2212-9391   ISSN 2212-9413 (electronic)
ISBN 978-3-319-35805-5   ISBN 978-3-319-07269-2 (eBook)
DOI 10.1007/978-3-319-07269-2
Springer Cham Heidelberg New York Dordrecht London

Printed on acid-free paper

Springer is part of Springer Science+Business Media (www.springer.com)

Preface

The spine represents both a vital central axis for the musculoskeletal system and a flexible protective shell surrounding the most important neural pathway in the body, the spinal cord. Spine-related diseases or conditions are common and cause a huge burden of morbidity and cost to society. Examples include degenerative disk disease, spinal stenosis, scoliosis, osteoporosis, herniated disks, fracture/ligamentous injury, infection, tumor, and spondyloarthropathy. Treatment varies with the disease entity and the clinical scenario can be nonspecific. As a result, imaging is often required to help make the diagnosis. Frequently obtained studies include plain radiographs, DXA, bone scans, CT, MR, ultrasound, and nuclear medicine. Computational methods play a steadily increasing role in improving speed, confidence, and accuracy in reaching a final diagnosis. Although there has been great progress in the development of computational methods for spine imaging over the recent years, there are a number of significant challenges in both methodology and clinical applications.

The goal of this workshop on "Computational Methods and Clinical Applications for Spine Imaging" was to bring together clinicians, computer scientists, and industrial vendors in the field of spine imaging, for reviewing the state-of-art techniques, sharing the novel and emerging analysis and visualization techniques, and discussing the clinical challenges and open problems in this rapidly growing field. We invited papers on all major aspects of problems related to spine imaging, including clinical applications of spine imaging, computer-aided diagnosis of spine conditions, computer Aided Detection of spine-related diseases, emerging computational imaging techniques for spinal diseases, fast 3D reconstruction of spine, feature extraction, multiscale analysis, pattern recognition, image enhancement of spine imaging, image-guided spine intervention and treatment, multimodal image registration and fusion for spine imaging, novel visualization techniques, segmentation techniques for spine imaging, statistical and geometric modeling for spine and vertebra, spine and vertebra localization.

Although being the first MICCAI workshop on this particular topic, we received many high quality submissions addressing many of the above-mentioned issues. All papers underwent a thorough double-blinded review with each paper being reviewed by three members of the program committee including workshop chairs. The program committee consisted of researchers who had actively contributed to the field of spine imaging in the past. From all submissions, we finally accepted 19 papers as oral presentations. The papers are organized into five parts according to the topics. The parts are Segmentation I (CT), Computer Aided Detection and Diagnosis, Quantitative Imaging, Segmentation II (MR) and Registration/Labeling.

In order to give deeper insights into the field and stimulate further ideas, we had invited lectures held during the workshop. We are very thankful to Tokumi Kanamura, Gabor Fichtinger, and Vipin Chaudhary for agreeing to give invited talks on the topic of clinical indications, image guided intervention, and commercialization.

We hope that with this workshop we have increased the attention toward this important and interesting field of computational spine imaging and would like to finally thank all contributors for their efforts in making this workshop possible. We especially thank the following institutes for their sponsorship: Journal of Computerized Medical Imaging and Graphics, GE Healthcare, Digital Imaging group of London, Philips Research, and National Institutes of Health.

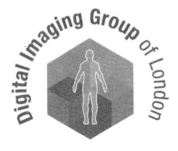

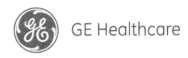

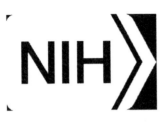

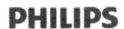

Jianhua Yao
Tobias Klinder
Aly A. Farag
Shuo Li

Workshop Organization

Organizing Committee

Jianhua Yao, *National Institutes of Health, USA*
Tobias Klinder, *Philips Research, Germany*
Aly A. Farag, *University of Louisville, USA*
Shuo Li, *GE Healthcare and University of Western Ontario, Canada*

Clinical Advisory

Gregory J. Garvin, *St. Joseph's Health Care, Canada*
KengYeow Tay, *Victoria Hospital, Canada*
Joseph E. Burns, *University of California, Irvine, USA*
Ronald M. Summers, *National Institutes of Health, USA*

Program Committee

Ulas Bagci, *National Institutes of Health, USA*
Li Bai, *University of Nottingham, UK*
Jonathan Biosvert, *National Research Council, Canada*
Xinjian Chen, *Soochow University, China*
Ananda Chowdhury, *Jadavpur University, India*
Ben Glocker, *Microsoft Research, UK*
Seyed-Parsa Hojjat, *GE Healthcare, Canada*
Samuel Kadoury, *Ecole Polytechnique de Montreal, Canada*
Xiaofeng Liu, *GE Healthcare, USA*
Wai Kong Law Max, *GE Healthcare and University of Western Ontario, Canada*
Cristian Lorenz, *Philips Research*
Nikos Paragios, *Ecole Centrale de Paris, France*
Alberto Santamaria Pang, *GE Global Research*

Jay Tian, *Chinese Academy of Sciences, China*
Tomaž Vrtovec, *University of Ljubljana, Slovenia*
Michael Ward, *National Institutes of Health, USA*
Yiqiang Zhan, *Siemens Medical Solutions, USA*

Scientific Review Committee

Ulas Bagci, *National Institutes of Health, USA*
Jonathan Biosvert, *National Research Council, Canada*
Xinjian Chen, *Soochow University, China*
Ananda Chowdhary, *Jadavpur University, India*
Daniel Forsberg, *Linköping University, Sweden*
Ben Glocker, *Microsoft Research, UK*
Bulat Ibragimov, *University of Ljubljana, Slovenia*
Samuel Kadoury, *Ecole Polytechnique de Montreal, Canada*
Tobias Klinder, *Philips Research, Germany*
Poay Lim, *University of Nottingham, UK*
Jianfei Liu, *National Institutes of Health, USA*
Jiamin Liu, *National Institutes of Health, USA*
Yixun Liu, *National Institutes of Health, USA*
Xiaofeng Liu, *GE Healthcare, USA*
Meelis Lootus, *Oxford University, UK*
Le Lu, *National Institutes of Health, USA*
Wai Kong Law, *GE Healthcare and University of Western Ontario, Canada*
Ales Neubert, *University of Queensland, Australia*
Simon Pezold, *University of Basel, Switzerland*
Sovira Tan, *National Institutes of Health, USA*
Tomaž Vrtovec, *University of Ljubljana, Slovenia*
Qian Wang, *University of North Carolina at Chapel Hill, USA*
Shijun Wang, *National Institutes of Health, USA*
Tristan Whitmarsh, *University of Cambridge, UK*
Jianhua Yao, *National Institutes of Health, USA*
Yiqiang Zhang, *Siemens Medical Solutions, USA*
Weidong Zhang, *National Institutes of Health, USA*

Proceedings Editors

Jianhua Yao, *National Institutes of Health, USA*
Tobias Klinder, *Philips Research, Germany*
Shuo Li, *GE Healthcare and University of Western Ontario, Canada*

Contents

Part I
Segmentation I (CT)

Segmentation of Vertebrae from 3D Spine Images by Applying Concepts from Transportation and Game Theories

Bulat Ibragimov, Boštjan Likar, Franjo Pernuš and Tomaž Vrtovec

Abstract We describe a landmark-based three-dimensional (3D) segmentation framework, in which the shape representation of the object of interest is based on concepts from transportation theory. Landmark-based shape representation relies on a premise that considering spatial relationships for every pair of landmarks is redundant, therefore landmarks are first separated into clusters. Landmarks within each cluster form a complete graph of connections, while landmarks within any two clusters are connected in a one-to-one manner by applying a concept from transportation theory called the optimal assignment. The resulting optimal assignment-based shape representation captures the most descriptive shape properties and therefore represents an adequate balance among rigidity, elasticity and computational complexity, and is combined with a 3D landmark detection algorithm that is based on concepts from game theory. The framework was applied to segment 50 lumbar vertebrae from 3D computed tomography images, and the resulting symmetric surface distance of 0.76 ± 0.10 mm and Dice coefficient of 93.5 ± 1.0 % indicate that accurate segmentation can be obtained by the described framework. Moreover, when compared to the complete graph, the computational time was reduced by a factor of approximately nine in the case of optimal assignment-based shape representation.

B. Ibragimov (✉) · B. Likar · F. Pernuš · T. Vrtovec
Faculty of Electrical Engineering, University of Ljubljana, Tržaška cesta 25,
SI-1000 Ljubljana, Slovenia
e-mail: bulat.ibragimov@fe.uni-lj.si

B. Likar
e-mail: bostjan.likar@fe.uni-lj.si

F. Pernuš
e-mail: franjo.pernus@fe.uni-lj.si

T. Vrtovec
e-mail: tomaz.vrtovec@fe.uni-lj.si

J. Yao et al. (eds.), *Computational Methods and Clinical Applications
for Spine Imaging*, Lecture Notes in Computational Vision and Biomechanics 17,
DOI: 10.1007/978-3-319-07269-2_1, © Springer International Publishing Switzerland 2014

1 Introduction

Segmentation of vertebrae is among the most challenging segmentation problems, as vertebrae are highly articulated structures, consisting of the vertebral body, pedicles and processes. As a result, the application of unsupervised segmentation approaches is limited, however, supervised segmentation approaches that require prior modeling of vertebral structures were already successfully applied, especially in the case of three-dimensional (3D) spine images [1–7]. For the segmentation of vertebral and also other anatomical structures, shape modeling has been mostly driven by active shape models (ASM) [8] and active appearance models (AAM) [9]. However, if the distance between the initial model and the object of interest is too large, model optimization may lead to an incorrect solution that is locally but not globally optimal. Moreover, intensities and shapes are generally treated separately and independently. To overcome these shortcomings, landmark-based segmentation methods, where the object of interest is described by intensity and shape properties of landmarks and connections among these landmarks, have been proposed [10–12]. However, methods that were originally developed for two-dimensional (2D) images cannot be directly applied to 3D images, because a considerably larger number of landmarks is required to accurately capture the shape of the object of interest in 3D. If the number of landmarks increases linearly, the number of connections among landmarks exhibits a quadratic growth, which is reflected in the computational complexity. In the case the shape is represented by a complete set of connections among landmarks (i.e. a complete graph), the resulting shape representation is strong and prevents non-plausible shape deformations in 2D, but may at the same time limit the shape elasticity in 3D. A balance among computational complexity, rigidity and elasticity may be obtained by reducing the complete set of connections [13], and the more recent approaches combined statistical properties of individual connections, defining local shape properties, and of the complete set of connections, defining global shape properties [11, 14]. Despite considerable improvements, existing approaches often result in a discriminative degree of connections for different landmarks, i.e. the number of connections established for different landmarks varies. In practice, this usually reflects in a high degree of connections for few landmarks and a low degree for most landmarks, which may lead to errors in landmark detection and formation of non-plausible shapes.

In this paper, we combine a non-discriminative landmark-based shape representation [15] with a landmark-based segmentation framework [12] and extend its application from 2D to 3D image segmentation (Fig. 1). The introduced 3D shape representation is based on concepts from transportation theory [16], and is integrated with a landmark-based detection in 3D that relies on concepts from game theory [17]. The resulting framework was validated for segmentation of lumbar vertebrae from 3D computed tomography (CT) spine images.

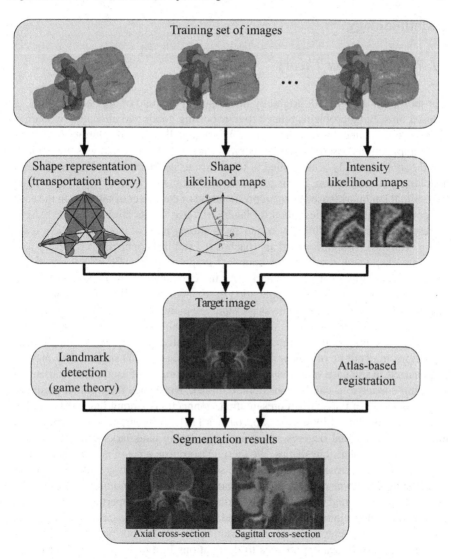

Fig. 1 An overview of the proposed segmentation framework. The 3D shape representation of the object of interest is determined by connections among landmarks that are established according to the optimal assignment, a special case of transportation theory. The shape and intensity likelihood maps are also computed for landmarks in images from the training set, and together with the shape representation used to guide landmark detection in the target image, which is based on concepts from game theory. The resulting landmarks in the target image are combined with an atlas-based image registration that combines landmarks and pre-segmented surfaces of the object of interest in the training set of images with landmarks in the target image to generate the final segmentation results in 3D

2 Methodology

2.1 Transportation Theory

Transportation theory [16], originally developed in the field of applied economy, is focused on solving problems related to transporting goods and allocating resources between sources and destinations, and provides globally optimal solutions for a variety of applications based on graph theory. In the field of image analysis, transportation theory has already been applied to solve various problems related to information matching and comparison. In this paper, we apply transportation theory to determine the optimal landmark-based shape representation of the object of interest. In the case the object of interest is described by landmarks $p \in \mathcal{P}$, its landmark-based shape representation can be defined by connections among pairs of landmarks $\forall p, q \in \mathcal{P}$; $p \neq q$. The most straightforward approach is to establish connections for every pair of landmarks, which results in the complete graph of $\frac{1}{2}|\mathcal{P}|(|\mathcal{P}| - 1)$ connections, where $|\mathcal{P}|$ is the number of landmarks. As the complete graph-based shape representation is relatively rigid, its application in segmentation will in general not result in non-plausible shapes, but some shapes that are plausible may not be detected due to its limited elasticity. Because a connection is established for every pair of landmarks, the resulting shape representation is also relatively complex. Although these limitations may not be of utmost importance in the case of 2D shapes, they may be emphasized in the case of 3D shapes, where the number of landmarks and corresponding connections can be considerably larger. To balance the rigidity, elasticity and complexity of the shape representation, connections among landmarks can be selectively established by various approaches [13]. However, existing approaches may result in unequal degrees of connections among landmarks (Fig. 2a), which may lead to non-plausible shapes. We therefore propose a novel non-discriminative statistical shape representation, where we selectively establish connections and, at the same time, enforce equal degrees of connections among landmarks. The process of establishing optimal connections is guided by statistical properties of landmarks, learned from the training set of images and then applied to the target image, and is observed from the perspective of transportation theory. For our purpose, we exploit a special case of allocating sources to destinations in a one-to-one manner called the optimal assignment, because it has several computationally effective solutions, e.g. the Hungarian algorithm [18].

2.2 Game Theory

Game theory [17] is a discipline that studies the behavior of decision makers, who play a game by making decisions that impact one another. A game is a set of rules for playing, and a play is a specific combination of these rules that occurs when each player (i.e. the decision maker) chooses a strategy (i.e. a decision as an admissible behavior of the decision maker) so that it maximizes his payoff (i.e. the benefit gained

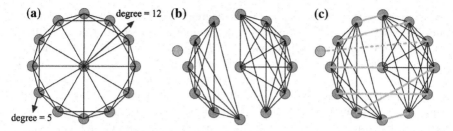

Fig. 2 a A shape representation consisting of 13 landmarks with unequal degrees of connections. **b** Separation of landmarks into two clusters of 6 and 7 landmarks (note that the cardinality of clusters is equalized by a pseudo-landmark). Intra-cluster connections are established as complete graphs. **c** Optimal assignment-based shape representation, consisting of intra-cluster and also inter-cluster connections (in *green*), established by optimal assignment among landmarks in the two clusters

according to the behavior of other players). In non-cooperative games, each player acts independently and aims to maximize his payoff regardless of payoffs gained by other players, while in cooperative games, players can join into coalitions (the grand coalition joins all players) and aim to maximize their joint payoff. In this paper, we apply game theory to detect the optimal position of landmarks that describe the object of interest. Landmark detection is considered as a game where landmarks are players, landmark candidate points are strategies, and likelihoods that each candidate point represents a landmark are payoffs [12]. As players (i.e. landmarks) can simultaneously participate in maximizing their joint payoffs (i.e. cumulative likelihoods) through the corresponding strategies (i.e. landmark candidate points), landmark detection in the target image can be represented as a cooperative game with the grand coalition and solved by maximizing the joint payoff ϑ^*:

$$\vartheta^* (\mathcal{P}, \mathcal{S}, \mathcal{W}) = \arg\max_{\omega} \left(\sum_{p \in \mathcal{P}} w_p \right), \tag{1}$$

where $\mathcal{P}$ and $\mathcal{S} = \mathcal{S}_p \cup \mathcal{S}_q \cup \ldots$ are, respectively, sets of landmarks and landmark candidate points, w_p is the payoff for landmark $p \in \mathcal{P}$, $\omega = \{w_p, w_q, \ldots\}$ is an admissible combination of payoffs, and $\mathcal{W} = \{W_{p,q}; \forall p, q \in \mathcal{P}, p \neq q\}$ is the payoff matrix that consists of matrices $W_{p,q}$ of partial payoffs for each pair of landmarks $p, q \in \mathcal{P}$. The element of $W_{p,q}$ at location (s_p, s_q) represents the partial payoff of landmark p if landmarks p and q are represented by, respectively, candidate points $s_p \in \mathcal{S}_p$ and $s_q \in \mathcal{S}_q$.

2.3 Optimal Assignment-Based 3D Shape Representation

Let the object of interest be in each image from the training set T annotated by corresponding landmarks $p \in \mathcal{P}$. The application of optimal assignment to all landmarks would result in a weak shape representation, because every landmark would be connected to only one other landmark (i.e. the degree of connections would be equal to one). To avoid such situation, we first divide landmarks into L clusters, each with the same number of landmarks $|\mathcal{C}|$, so that $|\mathcal{P}| \approx L |\mathcal{C}|$ (if the same cardinality cannot be achieved for every cluster, it is equalized by introducing pseudo-landmarks). Landmarks within each ith cluster are connected by a complete graph $\mathcal{G}_i^*$, resulting in intra-cluster connections (Fig. 2b). For all clusters, the total number of intra-cluster connections is therefore $\frac{1}{2}L |\mathcal{C}| (|\mathcal{C}| - 1)$. Moreover, each landmark from ith cluster is connected to exactly one landmark from every other jth cluster, resulting in inter-cluster connections (Fig. 2c). For all clusters, the total number of inter-cluster connections is therefore $\frac{1}{2} |\mathcal{P}| (L - 1)$. The inter-cluster connections are defined by the optimal assignment $\mathcal{A}_{i,j}^*$ that corresponds to the maximal total benefit of a shape representation [18]:

$$
\mathcal{A}_{i,j}^* = \arg\max_{\mathfrak{a} \in \mathcal{A}_{i,j}} \left(\sum_{p \in \mathcal{C}_i} u \left(D_{p,\mathfrak{a}(p)}, \Phi_{p,\mathfrak{a}(p)}, \Theta_{p,\mathfrak{a}(p)} \right) \right) ; \quad \begin{array}{l} i, j = 1, \ldots, L; \\ i \neq j, \end{array} \quad (2)
$$

where $\mathcal{A}_{i,j}$ is the set of all possible one-to-one assignments among landmarks between ith and jth cluster in the form of bijections $i \to j$, $\mathfrak{a}(p)$ is the landmark from jth cluster that is assigned to landmark p from ith cluster by bijection $\mathfrak{a} \in \mathcal{A}_{i,j}$, and $u(\cdot)$ is a linear function that is composed of probability distributions of distances $D_{p,\mathfrak{a}(p)}$, azimuth angles $\Phi_{p,\mathfrak{a}(p)}$ and polar angles $\Theta_{p,\mathfrak{a}(p)}$. These probability distributions describe the 3D spatial relationships, observed in the spherical coordinate system, between any two landmarks $p, q \in \mathcal{P}$ that occur in images from the training set and are computed as:

$$
X_{p,q} \left(x_{p,q}, \sigma_X, x \right) = \sum_{n \in T} \frac{1}{\sigma_X} \exp\left(-\frac{\left(x_{p,q}(n) - x \right)^2}{2\sigma_X^2} \right), \quad (3)
$$

where $x_{p,q}(n)$ is the feature value for landmarks p and q in the nth image from the training set T, x is an arbitrary feature value ($0 \leq x \leq x_{\max}$), and σ_X is a predefined constant that tunes the sensitivity of the distribution to feature value variations. The resulting distance, azimuth angle and polar angle distributions are therefore, respectively, $D_{p,q}(d) = X_{p,q}(d_{p,q}, \sigma_D, d)$, $\Phi_{p,q}(\varphi) = X_{p,q}(\varphi_{p,q}, \sigma_\Phi, \varphi)$ and $\Theta_{p,q}(\theta) = X_{p,q}(\theta_{p,q}, \sigma_\Theta, \theta)$, where $d_{p,q}$ is the distance, $\varphi_{p,q}$ is the azimuth angle, and $\theta_{p,q}$ is the polar angle between landmarks p and q.

The resulting optimal assignment $\mathcal{A}_{i,j}^*$ between ith and jth cluster defines the set $\{1_{p,q}\}$ of indicator functions for landmarks p from ith cluster and landmarks q from jth cluster. Each indicator function $1_{p,q}$ equals 1 if the inter-cluster connection between landmarks p and q was established, and 0 otherwise. On the other hand, for intra-cluster connections in ith cluster that result from $\mathcal{G}_i^*$, the indicator function $1_{p,q}$ always equals 1, as the connections form a complete graph.

2.4 Landmark-Based 3D Image Segmentation

Landmark-based image segmentation is the problem of finding landmarks that define the object of interest in an unknown target image, and one of the options is to exploit the statistical information of shape representations in the annotated training set of images. We first extract the statistical information from the training set of images in the form of intensity and shape likelihood maps, then use the intensity likelihood maps to identify landmark candidate points, and finally use both intensity and shape likelihood maps to detect the combination of optimal candidate points that represents landmarks in the target image.

For each corresponding landmark $p \in \mathcal{P}$ we first compute the mean image intensity μ_p at every point in its neighborhood across the images in the training set T. At location v in the target image, which is a candidate for landmark p, the intensity likelihood map $f_p(v)$ is computed as a cross-correlation between μ_p and image intensities at every point in the neighborhood of v. The set $\mathcal{S}_p$ of M candidate points for landmark p in the target image is obtained by selecting points at locations of M largest maxima of f_p (Fig. 3a). The shape likelihood map $g_{p,q}$ is defined as a linear combination of the distance ($D_{p,q}$), azimuth angle ($\Phi_{p,q}$) and polar angle ($\Theta_{p,q}$) probability distributions (Eq. 3):

$$g_{p,q}(d, \varphi, \theta, \Delta, \Upsilon, \Omega) = \lambda_1 D_{p,q}(\Delta \cdot d) + \lambda_2 \Phi_{p,q}(\varphi + \Upsilon) + \lambda_3 \Theta_{p,q}(\theta + \Omega) \quad (4)$$

and therefore represents the shape variations for landmarks p and q in images from the training set T. The parameters $\mathcal{R} = \{\Delta, \Upsilon, \Omega\}$ serve to additionally scale and rotate the system of landmarks p and q, and therefore compensate for an eventual global scaling and rotation of the object of interest. The parameters λ_i weight the contribution of individual probability distributions; $\sum_{i=1}^{3} \lambda_i = 1, \forall i: \lambda_i \geq 0$.

The resulting intensity (f_p) and shape ($g_{p,q}$) likelihood maps, and the optimal assignment-based shape representation ($\mathcal{G}^* \cup \mathcal{A}^*$) are combined with an existing landmark-based image segmentation framework [12] that relies on concepts from game theory [17]. The partial payoff (Eq. 1) of landmark p if landmarks p and q are represented by, respectively, candidate points $s_p \in \mathcal{S}_p$ and $s_q \in \mathcal{S}_q$ is defined as:

$$W_{p,q}(s_p, s_q, \mathcal{R}) = (1 - \tau) f_p(v_{s_p}) + \tau g_{p,q}\left(d_{s_p,s_q}, \varphi_{s_p,s_q}, \theta_{s_p,s_q}, \mathcal{R}\right), \quad (5)$$

where v_{s_p} is the location of s_p in the target image, d_{s_p,s_q}, φ_{s_p,s_q} and θ_{s_p,s_q} are, respectively, the distance, azimuth angle and polar angle between s_p and s_q in the target image, $\mathcal{R} = \{\Delta, \Upsilon, \Omega\}$ are the parameters that compensate for the global scaling and rotation of the object of interest (Eq. 4), and τ weights the contribution of the intensity and shape likelihood maps; $0 \leq \tau \leq 1$.

The cooperative game with the grand coalition is, in terms of combinatorial optimization, a relatively complex problem. However, a locally optimal combination of candidate points $\sigma^* = \{s_p^*, s_q^*, \ldots\}$ can be obtained by an iterative optimiza-

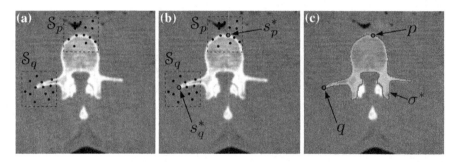

Fig. 3 The proposed landmark-based segmentation of the L1 vertebra, shown in an axial CT cross-section. **a** Candidate points for landmarks p and q form the corresponding sets $\mathcal{S}_p$ and $\mathcal{S}_q$. **b** The optimal candidate points s_p^* and s_q^* are found by the game-theoretic landmark detection. **c** The set of optimal candidate points σ^* represents landmarks that define the boundary of the object of interest

tion algorithm [12]. According to Eqs. 1 and 5, and by considering the optimal assignment-based shape representation, we define the total payoff ψ as:

$$\psi(q, s_q, {}^k\mathcal{P}, {}^k\mathcal{S}, \mathcal{W}, \mathcal{R}) = \sum_{i \in {}^k\mathcal{P}} \sum_{\substack{j \in {}^k\mathcal{P} \\ j \neq i}} 1_{i,j} W_{i,j}(s_i, s_j, \mathcal{R}) \qquad (6)$$

$$+ \sum_{i \in {}^k\mathcal{P}} 1_{i,q} W_{i,q}(s_i, s_q, \mathcal{R})$$

$$+ \sum_{j \in {}^k\mathcal{P}} 1_{q,j} W_{q,j}(s_q, s_j, \mathcal{R}),$$

where ${}^k\mathcal{P}$ is an observed subset of landmarks without landmark q; ${}^k\mathcal{P} \subset \mathcal{P}\backslash\{q\}$, ${}^k\mathcal{S}$ is the combination of optimal candidate points that correspond to landmarks in ${}^k\mathcal{P}$ (each landmark is associated with exactly one optimal candidate point), $1_{p,q}$ is the indicator function obtained from the optimal assignment $\mathcal{G}^* \cup \mathcal{A}^*$, and k denotes the current configuration of sets ${}^k\mathcal{P}$ and ${}^k\mathcal{S}$ that are associated with the iteration of the optimization algorithm. By maximizing the above described total payoff ψ, the optimal combination of candidate points $\sigma^* = \{s_p^*, s_q^*, \ldots\}$ can be detected in polynomial time.

The obtained combination of optimal candidate points $\sigma^* = \{s_p^*, s_q^*, \ldots\}$ represents landmarks in the target image that correspond to $\mathcal{P} = \{p, q, \ldots\}$. In the case the object of interest is, in each image from the training set, segmented in the form of a binary mask, its 3D segmentation in the target image can be achieved by atlasing these binary masks from images in the training set to the target image. For each image in the training set, landmarks are first non-rigidly registered to the obtained combination of optimal candidate points σ^*, and the resulting transformation is used to propagate the corresponding binary mask to the target image. The propagated and transformed binary masks of all images in the training set are accumulated in the target image, and voxels for which the overlap in accumulated binary masks exceeds a predefined threshold are selected as the final 3D segmentation of the object of interest.

3 Experiments and Results

The proposed framework was applied to segment 50 vertebrae that were obtained from 10 CT lumbar spine images with in-plane voxel size of 0.282–0.791 mm and slice thickness of 0.725–1.530 mm. Vertebrae at each segment (i.e. L1 to L5) were first manually segmented, and the resulting 10 binary masks were non-rigidly registered [19] to obtain surface correspondences. The obtained transformation fields were then used to propagate $|\mathcal{P}| = 300$ landmarks, which were evenly distributed on the surface of one binary mask, to the remaining nine binary masks, resulting in sets of corresponding landmarks. By applying the k-means algorithm, landmarks were divided into $L = 18$ clusters, each with $|\mathcal{C}| \approx \sqrt{|\mathcal{P}|} = 17$ landmarks (pseudo-landmarks were added to corresponding clusters to equalize the number of landmarks in each cluster, therefore $|\mathcal{P}| \to |\mathcal{P}'| = L\,|\mathcal{C}| = 306$). Within each cluster, connections were established as complete graphs, amounting to $\frac{1}{2}L\,|\mathcal{C}|\,(|\mathcal{C}| - 1) = 2{,}448$ intra-cluster connections. Between any pair of clusters, connections were established by optimal assignment, amounting to $\frac{1}{2}|\mathcal{P}'|\,(L - 1) = 2{,}601$ inter-cluster connections. The total number of connections in the resulting optimal assignment-based representation was therefore $2{,}448 + 2601 = 5{,}049$, which is approximately nine times less than in the case of the complete graph-based shape representation with $\frac{1}{2}|\mathcal{P}|\,(|\mathcal{P}| - 1) = 44{,}850$ connections. The remaining parameters of the framework were set to $u(\cdot) = \frac{1}{|T|}\sum_{n \in T} d_{p,q}(n)$ (the linear function in Eq. 2), $\sigma_D = 15$ mm and $\sigma_\Phi = \sigma_\Theta = 15°$ (parameters of probability distributions in Eq. 3), $M = 30$ (the number of candidate points for each landmark, obtained on the basis of $11 \times 11 \times 11$ mm large neighborhoods), $\lambda_1 = 0.7$, $\lambda_2 = 0.2$ and $\lambda_3 = 0.1$ (weights of the contribution of probability distributions in Eq. 4), $\tau = 0.9$ (weight of the contribution of the intensity and shape likelihood map in Eq. 5), and 50 % threshold for the overlap in the binary mask accumulation. These parameter values were determined experimentally by observing their impact on the final segmentation, however, they may be further tuned for a specific application.

The proposed framework was implemented in C++ without any code optimization, and executed on a personal computer with Intel Core i7 processor at 2.8 GHz and 8 GB of memory without any hardware-assisted acceleration. The segmentation performance was validated by leave-one-out experiments, one for each vertebral segment, i.e. the framework was iteratively trained on nine vertebrae and applied to segment the remaining vertebra of the same segment. The results are for individual vertebral segments presented in Table 1 in terms of symmetric surface distance δ and Dice coefficient κ, measured against reference binary masks that were obtained by manual segmentation, and in terms of computational time t. For all vertebral segments,

Table 1 Lumbar vertebra segmentation results in terms of symmetric surface distance δ, Dice coefficient κ and computational time t, reported as mean $\pm$ standard deviation (generation of intensity likelihood maps requires 4–6 min per vertebra and is not included)

Vertebral segment	Optimal assignment-based shape representation (5,049 connections)			Complete graph-based shape representation (44,850 connections)		
	δ (mm)	κ (%)	t (s)	δ (mm)	κ (%)	t (s)
L1	0.71 ± 0.07	93.9 ± 0.6	81 ± 5	0.78 ± 0.11	93.5 ± 0.7	709 ± 28
L2	0.73 ± 0.07	94.1 ± 0.5	66 ± 4	0.75 ± 0.08	93.6 ± 0.5	596 ± 17
L3	0.76 ± 0.08	93.8 ± 0.5	68 ± 4	0.81 ± 0.10	93.2 ± 0.7	612 ± 18
L4	0.81 ± 0.15	92.8 ± 1.4	90 ± 2	0.86 ± 0.15	92.1 ± 1.4	804 ± 10
L5	0.78 ± 0.11	92.9 ± 1.6	92 ± 3	0.82 ± 0.16	91.9 ± 2.0	811 ± 12

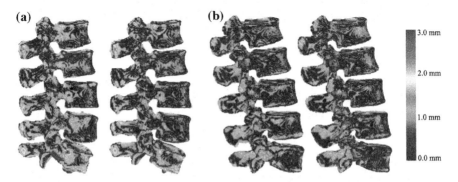

Fig. 4 Segmentation results for two selected images of lumbar vertebrae (**a, b**), obtained by applying the complete graph-based (*left*) and optimal assignment-based (*right*) shape representation (the colormap encodes the symmetric surface distance δ against the corresponding reference binary masks)

the mean values were $\delta = 0.76 \pm 0.10$ mm, $\kappa = 93.5 \pm 1.0\%$ and $t = 79 \pm 4$ s for the optimal assignment-based shape representation, and $\delta = 0.80 \pm 0.12$ mm, $\kappa = 92.9 \pm 1.2\%$ and $t = 706 \pm 18$ s for the complete graph-based shape representation. The results show that accurate segmentation can be obtained both by the optimal assignment-based and complete graph-based shape representation (Fig. 4). However, as the number of connections was considerably lower in the case of the optimal assignment-based shape representation, the computational time was reduced by a factor of approximately nine, i.e. proportionally to the number of established connections. At the same time, the segmentation accuracy was improved when compared to the complete graph-based shape representation, which indicates that an adequate balance among rigidity, elasticity and complexity was achieved by introducing the optimal assignment-based shape representation.

4 Discussion and Conclusion

In this paper, we presented a framework for landmark-based 3D image segmentation that combines a landmark-based 3D shape representation with a reduced number of connections among landmarks, determined by using concepts from transportation theory, and a landmark detection algorithm, which relies on concepts from game theory. The process of landmark detection results in a set of optimal candidate points for landmarks that define the shape of the object of interest, and were obtained by simultaneously considering the intensity likelihood maps of individual landmarks and the shape likelihood maps of selected connections among landmarks with the largest shape representativeness. The landmarks were divided into clusters, and for every cluster, connections among landmarks were established in the form of complete graphs, while for every pair of clusters, connections among landmarks were established by optimally assigning landmarks between clusters in a one-to-one manner. The resulting optimal assignment-based shape representation was a combination of intra-cluster connections that captured the shape of local regions, and inter-cluster connections that captured the global shape of the object of interest. By replacing the complete graph-based shape representation with the optimal assignment-based shape representation, segmentation became less prone to non-plausible deformations, the elasticity of the shape was enabled, and the computational complexity was considerably reduced. The proposed framework does not depend on any initialization and all possible combinations of candidate points were simultaneously taken into account, therefore it was more likely to converge to the globally optimal solution. The performance of the framework was evaluated for segmentation of lumbar vertebrae from CT images. The obtained mean symmetric surface distance of $\delta = 0.76$ mm is equal to the lowest value presented in the literature that can be found in the work of Klinder et al. [3], while the obtained Dice coefficient of $\kappa = 93.5$ % is comparable to the lowest value presented in the literature, which equals 92.5 % in the work of Kadoury et al. [6, 7]. The performance of the proposed framework is therefore similar to the existing approaches, however, they were validated on different databases and, as such, segmentation results cannot be directly compared.

Nevertheless, for a thorough evaluation of the segmentation performance, the proposed framework needs to be validated on a larger training set of images, which has to include also images of diseased or pathological vertebrae, e.g. wedged vertebrae that may occur in the case of scoliosis or fractured vertebrae that may occur due to osteoporosis. On the other hand, the described framework is formulated in a general form, and is therefore not limited to segmentation of vertebrae from CT images, but may be easily adapted to other anatomical structures and imaging modalities. As such, it can be applied to a variety of segmentation problems where it is possible to effectively describe the shape of the object of interest by landmarks.

Acknowledgments This work has been supported by the Slovenian Research Agency under grants P2-0232, J7-2264, L2-7381, and L2-2023.

References

1. Kim, Y., Kim, D.: A fully automatic vertebra segmentation method using 3D deformable fences. Comput. Med. Imaging Graph. **33**(5), 343–352 (2009)
2. Huang, S.-H., Chu, Y.-H., Lai, S.-H., Novak, C.L.: Learning-based vertebra detection and iterative normalized-cut segmentation for spinal MRI. IEEE Trans. Med. Imaging **28**(10), 1595–1605 (2009)
3. Klinder, T., Ostermann, J., Ehm, M., Franz, A., Kneser, R., Lorenz, C.: Automated model-based vertebra detection, identification, and segmentation in CT images. Med. Image Anal. **13**(3), 471–482 (2009)
4. Ma, J., Lu, L., Zhan, Y., Zhou, X., Salganicoff, M., Krishnan, A.: Hierarchical segmentation and identification of thoracic vertebra using learning-based edge detection and coarse-to-fine deformable model. In; Proceedings of the 13th International Conference on Medical Image Computing and Computer-Assisted Intervention (MICCAI 2010), 20–24 Sept, Beijing. Lecture Notes in Computer Science, vol. 6361, pp. 19–27 (2010)
5. Štern, D., Likar, B., Pernuš, F., Vrtovec, T.: Parametric modelling and segmentation of vertebral bodies in 3D CT and MR spine images. Phys. Med. Biol. **56**(23), 7505–7522 (2011)
6. Kadoury, S., Labelle, H., Paragios, N.: Automatic inference of articulated spine models in CT images using high-order Markov random fields. Med. Image Anal. **15**(4), 426–437 (2011)
7. Kadoury, S., Labelle, H., Paragios, N.: Spine segmentation in medical images using manifold embeddings and higher-order MRFs. IEEE Trams. Med. Imaging **32**(7), 1227–1238 (2013)
8. Cootes, T., Taylor, C., Cooper, D., Graham, J.: Active shape models-their training and application. Comput. Vis. Image Underst. **61**(1), 38–59 (1995)
9. Cootes, T., Edwards, G., Taylor, C.: Active appearance models. IEEE Trans. Pattern Anal. **23**(6), 681–685 (2001)
10. Seghers, D., Loeckx, D., Maes, F., Vandermeulen, D., Suetens, P.: Minimal shape and intensity cost path segmentation. IEEE Ttans. Med. Imaging **26**(8), 1115–1129 (2007)
11. Besbes, A., Paragios, N.: Landmark-based segmentation of lungs while handling partial correspondences using sparse graph-based priors. In: Proceedings of the 2011 IEEE International Symposium on Biomedical Imaging: From Nano to Macro, 30 Mar–2 Apr, Chicago, pp. 989–995 (2011)
12. Ibragimov, B., Likar, B., Pernuš, F., Vrtovec, T.: A game-theoretic framework for landmark-based image segmentation. IEEE Trans. Med. Imaging **31**(9), 1761–1776 (2012)
13. Sawada, Y., Hontani, H.: A study on graphical model structure for representing statistical shape model of point distribution model. In: Proceedings of the 15th International Conference on Medical Image Computing and Computer-Assisted Intervention (MICCAI 2012), 1–5 Oct, Nice. Lecture Notes in Computer Science, vol. 7511, pp. 470–477 (2012)
14. Friedman, J., Hastie, T., Tibshirani, R.: Sparse inverse covariance estimation with the graphical lasso. Biostatistics **9**(3), 432–441 (2008)
15. Ibragimov, B., Pernuš, F., Likar, B., Vrtovec, T.: Statistical shape representation with landmark clustering by solving the assignment problem. In: Proceedings of the SPIE Medical Imaging 2013: Image Processing Conference, 9–14 Feb, Lake Buena Vista, vol. 8669, pp. 86690E (2013)
16. Schrijver, A.: Combinatorial optimization: polyhedra and efficiency. Springer, Berlin (2003)
17. von Neumann, J., Morgenstern, O.: Theory of games and economic behavior. Princeton University Press (1944)
18. Kuhn, H.W.: The Hungarian method for the assignment problem. In: Jünger, M. et al. (Eds.), 50 Years of Integer Programming 1958–2008. Springer, Berlin, pp. 29–47 (2010)
19. Kroon, D.-J.: B-spline grid, image and point based registration. http://www.mathworks.com/matlabcentral/fileexchange/20057 (2012). Accessed via 5 Nov 2012

Automatic and Reliable Segmentation of Spinal Canals in Low-Resolution, Low-Contrast CT Images

Qian Wang, Le Lu, Dijia Wu, Noha El-Zehiry, Dinggang Shen
and Kevin S. Zhou

Abstract Accurate segmentation of spinal canals in Computed Tomography (CT) images is an important task in many related studies. In this paper, we propose an automatic segmentation method and apply it to our highly challenging 110 datasets from the CT channel of PET-CT scans. We adapt the interactive random-walks (RW) segmentation algorithm to be fully automatic which is initialized with robust voxelwise classification using Haar features and probabilistic boosting tree. One-shot RW is able to estimate yet imperfect segmentation. We then refine the topology of the segmented spinal canal leading to improved seeds or boundary conditions of RW. Therefore, by iteratively optimizing the spinal canal topology and running RW segmentation, satisfactory segmentation results can be acquired within only a few iterations. Our experiments validate the capability of the proposed method with promising segmentation performance, even though the resolution and the contrast of our datasets are low.

Q. Wang (✉)
Department of Computer Science, Department of Radiology and BRIC, University of North
Carolina at Chapel Hill, Chapel Hill, NC, USA
e-mail: qianwang@cs.unc.edu

L. Lu
Radiology and Imaging Science, National Institutes of Health (NIH) Clinical Center,
Bethesda, MD, USA
e-mail: le.lu@nih.gov

D. Wu · N. El-Zehiry · K. S. Zhou
Siemens Corporate Research, Princeton, NJ, USA
e-mail: dijia.wu@siemens.con

D. Shen
Department of Radiology and BRIC, University of North Carolina at Chapel Hill, Chapel
Hill, NC, USA
e-mail: dgshen@med.unc.edu

J. Yao et al. (eds.), *Computational Methods and Clinical Applications*
for Spine Imaging, Lecture Notes in Computational Vision and Biomechanics 17,
DOI: 10.1007/978-3-319-07269-2_2, © Springer International Publishing Switzerland 2014

(a)   (b)   (c)

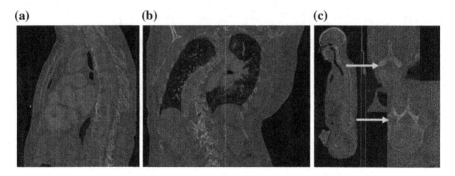

Fig. 1 Examples of datasets in our studies: **a** Sagittal view of restricted FOV near the chest area only; **b** Coronal view of disease-affected spine; **c** Sagittal view of full-body scan. Two additional transverse planes show that the spinal canal is not always contoured by bones

1 Introduction

To segment spinal canals is desirable in many studies because it facilitates analysis, diagnosis, and therapy planning related to spines. Segmentation of spinal canal provides helpful references to parcellate other anatomical structures and contributes to the understandings of full-body scans essentially [1]. Given spinal canal, it is much easier to delineate spinal cord, which is vulnerable to dosage tolerance and crucial for radiotherapy [2]. More previous works on spinal canal/cord focus on MR images, partly due to the better capability of MRI in rendering soft tissues. However, in this paper, we present an automatic method to segment spinal canals in low-resolution, low-contrast CT images. In particular, our highly diverse datasets are acquired from the CT channel in PET-CT and on pathological subjects. They are collected from eight different sites and vary significantly in Field-of-View (FOV), resolution, SNR, pathology, etc. Sagittal views of two typical datasets with different FOVs are shown in Fig. 1a, c, respectively. The coronal plane of another patient, whose spine twists due to diseases, is also provided in Fig. 1b. High variation and limited quality of the datasets have incurred additional difficulty in segmenting spinal canals.

Most spinal canal segmentation methods in the literature are semi-automatic [3–5], which require manual initializations or interactions. Archip et al. [2] present a fully automatic pipeline by parsing objects in a recursive manner. Specifically, body con-tour and bones are extracted first. Then region growing is employed to segment spinal canal on each slice independently. When the boundary of spinal canal is relatively weak as shown in top-right of Fig. 1c, this approach does not suffice and thus Snakes [6] is used to incorporate segmentation results from neighboring slices. Following similar top-down parcellation strategy, [7] uses watershed and graph search to segment spinal canals. However, this top-down parcellation depends on locating the spine column first to provide rough but important spatial reference, which can be nevertheless non-trivial.

Interactive segmentation has also developed rapidly and drawn many successes in past decades. By allowing users to define initial seeds, the interactive mechanism is able to understand image content better and generate improved segmentation results in the end. We refer readers to [8] for a comprehensive survey of interactive segmentation methods. Among them, random walks (RW) [9] has been widely applied in various studies. RW asks users to specify seeding voxels of different labels, and then assigns labels to non-seeding voxels by embedding the image into a graph and utilizing intensity similarity between voxels. Users can edit the placement of seeds in order to acquire more satisfactory results.

In this paper, we adapt the idea of interactive segmentation to form a fully automatic approach that segments spinal canals from CT images. Different from manually editing seeds in the interactive mode, our method refines the topology of the spinal canal and improves segmentation in the automatic and iterative manner. To start the automatic pipeline, we identify voxels that are inside the spinal canal according to their appearance features [10]. For convenience, we will denote the voxels inside the spinal canal as foreground, and background otherwise. Then the detected seeds are input to RW and produce the segmentation of foreground/background. Based on the tentative segmentation, we extract and further refine the topology of the spinal canal by considering both geometry and appearance constraints. Seeds are adjusted accordingly and fed back to RW for better segmentation. By iteratively applying this scheme, we are able to cascade several RW solvers and build a highly reliable method to segment spinal canals from CT images, even under challenging conditions.

Our method and its bottom-up design, significantly different from the top-down parcellation in other solutions, utilize both population-based appearance information and subject-specific geometry model. With limited training subjects, we are able to locate enough seeding voxels to initialize segmentation and iteratively improve the results by learning spinal canal topologies that vary significantly across patients. We will detail our method in Sect. 2, and show experimental results in Sect. 3.

2 Method

We treat segmenting spinal canal as a binary segmentation problem. Let p_x denote the probability of the voxel x being foreground (inside spinal canal) after voxel classification and $\bar{p}_x$ for background, respectively. In general, we have $p_x + \bar{p}_x = 1$ after normalization. The binary segmentation can be acquired by applying a threshold to p_x. Although shapes of spinal canals can vary significantly across the population, they are tubular structures in general. We start from a small set of foreground voxels with very high classification confidences. These voxels act as positive seeds in RW to generate conservative segmentation with relatively low sensitivity but also low false positives (FP). All foreground voxels are assumed to form a continuous and smooth anatomic topology, which refines the seed points in order to better approximate the structure of the spinal canal. Hence the sensitivity of the RW segmentation increases with the new seeds. By iteratively feeding the improved seeds to RW, we have successfully formed an automatic pipeline that yields satisfactory segmentation of spinal canals.

2.1 Voxelwise Classification

In order to identify highly reliable foreground voxels as positive seeds, we turn to voxelwise classification via supervised learning. We have manually annotated the medial lines of spinal canals on 20 CT datasets. Voxels exactly along the medial lines are sampled as foreground, while background candidates are obtained from a constant distance away to the medial lines. We further use 3D Haar features as voxel descriptors. With varying sizes of detection windows, an abundant collection of Haar features is efficiently computed for each voxel. The probabilistic boosting tree (PBT) classifiers are then trained with AdaBoost nodes [11]. We have cascaded multiple PBT classifiers that work in coarse-to-fine resolutions. In this way, we not only speed up the detection in early stage by reducing the number of samples, but also exploit features benefiting from higher scales of Haar wavelets in coarse resolution. Note that similar strategy is also successfully applied in other studies [10]. The well-performing foreground voxel confidence map (as well as the measuring color map) with respect to a training subject is displayed in Fig. 2a. However, when applied to a new testing dataset (e.g., Fig. 2c–d), the classifiers may suffer from both false negative (FN) and FP errors. For instance, an FP artifact is highlighted in Fig. 2b. Figure 2c shows discontinuity of foreground confidence due to FN errors. Since the purpose here is to preserve highly reliable foreground voxels only (i.e., Fig. 2d), we have adopted a high confidence threshold (>0.9) empirically to suppress most FP errors. The detection sensitivity will be subsequently improved as follows.

2.2 Random Walks

Similar to PBT-based classification, RW also produces voxelwise likelihoods of being foreground/background [9]. After users have specified foreground/background seeds, RW departs from a certain non-seeding voxel and calculates its probabilities to reach foreground and background seeds, as p_x and $\bar{p}_x$, respectively. Usually the non-seeding voxel x is assigned to foreground if $p_x > \bar{p}_x$. In the context of RW, the image is embedded into a graph where vertices correspond to individual voxels and edges link neighboring voxels. The weight w_{xy} of the edge e_{xy}, which measures the similarity between two neighboring voxels x and y, is defined as

$$w_{xy} = \exp(-\beta(I_x - I_y)^2), \tag{1}$$

where I_x and I_y represent intensities at two locations; β a positive constant. Assuming segmentation boundaries to be coincident with intensity changes, RW aims to

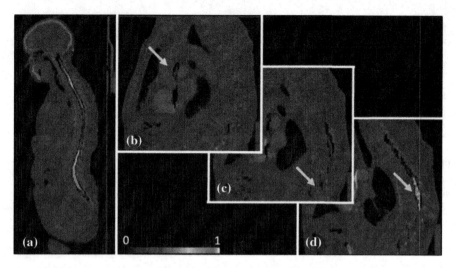

Fig. 2 Panel **a** shows the confidence map output by voxelwise classification on a *training* subject; panels **b–d** are for the voxelwise confidences of another *testing* dataset. Among them, FP errors and FN errors are highlighted in **b** and **c**, respectively. We use a high confidence threshold to preserve reliable foreground voxels only as in **d**

estimate p_x that satisfies to minimize the following energy term

$$E = \sum_{\forall e_{xy}} w_{xy}(p_x - p_y)^2. \tag{2}$$

To optimize the above is equivalent to solving a Dirichlet problem with boundary conditions defined by the seeds. Specifically, p_x is set to 1 if x is a foreground seed, and 0 for background. The calculated p_x incorporates spatial information of neighboring voxels, which differs from the independent voxelwise classification (Sect. 2.1).

The probability of each voxel in RW is associated with the paths from the voxel to seeds. Hence p_x is dependent not only on the weights of the edges forming the path, but also the length of each path. This potentially undermines RW that is sensitive to the seed locations. In the toy example of Fig. 3a, there are three vertical stripes. The intensity of the middle stripe is slightly different and approximates the spinal canal surrounded by other tissues in CT data. We highlight certain sections of stripe boundaries in very high intensity to simulate the existence of vertebra, whose presence can be discontinuous as in Fig. 1c. Foreground seeds and background seeds are colored in red and green, respectively. The calculated probability p_x in RW and the binary segmentation ($p_x > 0.5$) are shown. We observe from Fig. 3c that the segmented foreground falls into two segments undesirably. Though increasing the threshold on p_x and refining β to modify edge weights might improve the segmentation results, this becomes very ad-hoc. On the other hand, RW provides an interactive

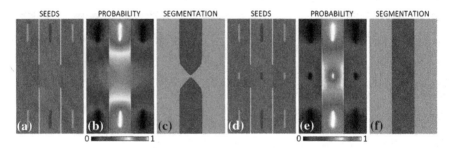

| SEEDS | PROBABILITY | SEGMENTATION | SEEDS | PROBABILITY | SEGMENTATION |

Fig. 3 With foreground seeds (*in red*) and background seeds (*in green*) **a**, the calculated probabilities **b** and the corresponding binary segmentation **c** are not satisfactory. However, by manually placing more seeds **d**, the segmentation results **e–f** are improved significantly

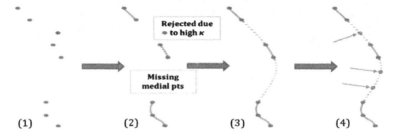

Fig. 4 Four sub-steps in refining the topology of the spinal canal include (*1*) estimating medial points; (*2*) determining medial segments; (*3*) calculating virtual medial segments (*in dotted curves*); and (*4*) placing more virtual medial points (*in purple*)

remedy by simply allowing users to place more seeds in proximity to the desired segmentation boundaries. The few additional seeds in Fig. 3d yield better discrepancy of foreground/background and lead to more satisfactory segmentation results (Fig. 3e–f).

2.3 Pipeline of Cascaded Random Walks

As mentioned above, we are able to identify seeds in voxel classification and feed them to RW for estimating segmentation. The initial segmented spinal canal usually breaks into several disconnected segments that imply high FN errors. This is because the initial seeds with high confidences from voxelwise classification are usually not sufficient to cover everywhere of the spinal canal.

Topology Refinement To refine and acquire complete segmentation, we introduce the topology constraints of the spinal canal to segmentation. Specifically, we use the medial line of the spinal canal to represent its topology. After calculating all segments of the medial line given the tentative segmentation, we interleave them into a single connected curve. Fig. 4 illustrates the four sub-steps to refine the topology of the spinal canal with regard to its medial line. Based on tentative segmentation (including outputs from voxelwise classification), we calculate the medial point of foreground voxels on each transverse slice in Fig. 4(1). The medial point is defined to have the least sum of distances to all other foreground voxels on each slice. Assuming that the medial line connects all medial points, we then connect the medial points into several segments in Fig. 4(2). The medial line may break into several segments since medial points can be missing. Also certain medial point would be rejected as outlier if it incurs too high curvature to the medial line. With all computed segments, we interleave them by filling gaps with smooth virtual segments (as dotted curves) in Fig. 4(3). Each virtual segment $c(s)$ minimizes $\int \|\nabla^2 c(s)\|^2 ds$ to keep smooth as $s \in [0, 1]$ for normalized arc-length. The stationary solution to the above holds when $\nabla^4 c(s) = 0$, and the Cauchy boundary conditions are defined by both two ends of the virtual segment as well as tangent directions at the ends. Though the numerical solution is non-unique, we apply the cubic Bézier curve for fast estimation of the virtual segment. For a certain virtual segment, we denote its ends as P_0 and P_3. An additional control point P_1 is placed so that the direction from P_0 to P_1 is identical to the tangent direction at P_0. Similarly, we can define P_2 according to P_3 and the associated tangent direction. We further require that the four control points are equally spaced. The virtual segment is $c(s) = (1-s)^3 P_0 + 3(1-s)^2 s P_1 + 3(1-s)s^2 P_2 + s^3 P_3$.

After predicting the virtual segment in Fig. 4(3), we finally place more virtual medial points along the virtual segment. Besides the subject-specific geometry constraints to keep the virtual segments smooth, we further incorporate appearance criterion in Fig. 4(4). Upon all existing medial points (red dots), we calculate their intensity mean and the standard deviation (STD). The univariate Gaussian intensity model allows us to examine whether a new voxel is highly possible to be foreground given its simple appearance value. In particular, we start from both two ends of each virtual segment, and admit virtual medial point (purple dot) if its intensity is within the single STD range of the intensity model. The process to admit virtual medial points aborts when a disqualified candidate has been encountered.

Seed Sampling After the topology of the spinal canal has been refined, we are able to provide better seeds for RW to use. All points along the refined medial line, including the newly admitted virtual ones, will act as foreground seeds. Moreover, we qualify more voxels as foreground seeds if (1) they have been classified as foreground in previous segmentation; (2) their intensities are within the single STD range of the appearance model introduced above; and (3) they are connected to the medial line via other foreground seeds. In this way, we have inherited previous segmentation in areas of high confidence, and saved computation since RW can simply treat them as boundary conditions. Surrounding voxels with high intensities will be regarded as bones and then counted as the background seeds.

Cascaded Random Walks By repeating the procedures above, we have cascaded several RW solvers in order to generate the final segmentation. The pipeline will terminate automatically when the topology of the spinal canal, or the length of the medial line, has become stable. Remaining medial segments that are isolated from others will then be excluded from the foreground, in that they usually reflect artifacts

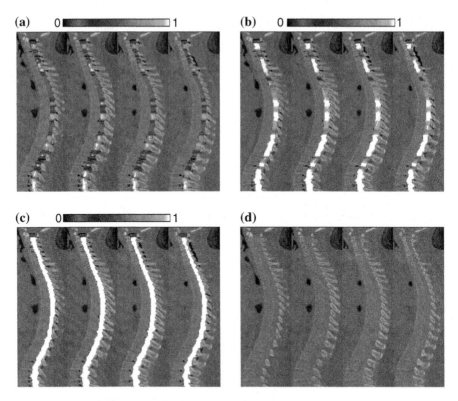

Fig. 5 Panels **a–c** show foreground probability on 4 consecutive slices of a certain subject output after the first, second, and the final (fourth) iteration, respectively. The binary segmentation in **d** is corresponding to the final probability in **c**

especially from legs. During the iterative refinement, we also allow the medial line to grow at its both ends and thus admit more virtual medial points. The growth can stop automatically at the tail and terminate in the head by limiting the maximal radial size of the spinal canal. In Fig. 5a, we show the foreground probability on four slices of a subject after the first iteration of our method. Improvement can be observed in Fig. 5b that shows the output after the second iteration. The final probability after the fourth iteration is shown in Fig. 5c, with the corresponding segmentation in Fig. 5d. The results above demonstrate that our method can efficiently utilize the topology of the spinal canal and generate satisfactory segmentation in the final.

3 Experimental Result

We have conducted a study on 110 individual images from eight medical sites, as the largest scale reported in the literature, to verify the capability of our method. The training data are not used for the sake of testing. Even though the image quality of our

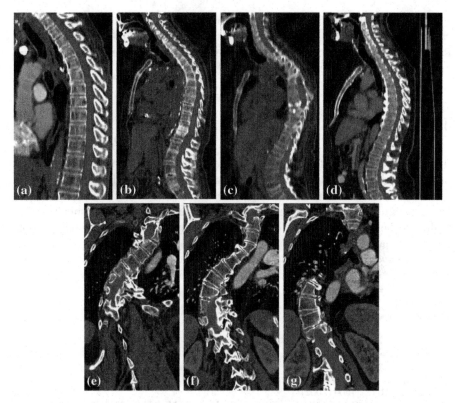

Fig. 6 Panels **a**–**d** show segmentation results (in sagittal views) on 4 randomly selected images. Coronal views of the segmentation results on an extreme case, whose spine twists due to diseases, are shown in **e**–**g**

data is low and the appearance variation is extremely high, we successfully generate good segmentation results on all datasets by our method with a fixed configuration. Sagittal views of segmentation results for 4 randomly selected subjects are shown in Fig. 6a–d, respectively. In Fig. 6e–g, we also show the segmentation result in 3 coronal slices for the extreme case in Fig. 1b. This patient is under influences from severe diseases, which cause an unusual twist to the spine. However, though the topology of the spinal canal under consideration is abnormal, our method is still capable to well segment the whole structure. All results above confirm that our method is robust in dealing with the challenging data.

We have further manually annotated 20 datasets for quantitative evaluation. For the manually delineated parts, the Dice overlapping ratio between the segmentation of our method and the ground truth reaches $92.79 \pm 1.55\%$. By visual inspection, robust and good segmentation results are achieved on all 110 datasets, especially including many highly pathological cases. Note that to deal with image data with severe pathologies is not addressed and validated in the previous literature [2–5, 7].

Our method achieves final segmentation in 2–5 iterations for all datasets, and typically costs 20–60 s per volume depending on the image size. With more sophisticated
RW method that is better designed for editing seeds [12], the speed performance of
our method can be further improved.

4 Discussion

In this work, an automatic method to segment spinal canals from low-quality CT
images is proposed. With initial seeds provided by PBT-based classification, we
introduce topology constraints into segmentation via RW. Our iterative optimization
has successfully enhanced the capability of RW in dealing with tubular spinal canals,
in that the boundary conditions can be improved to guarantee better segmentation
results. Our large-scale evaluation shows that the proposed method is highly accurate
and robust even if the datasets are very diverse and challenging.

References

1. Klinder, T., Ostermann, J., Ehm, M., Franz, A., Kneser, R., Lorenz, C.: Med. Image Anal.
   13(3), 471 (2009)
2. Archip, N., Erard, P.J., Egmont-Petersen, M., Haefliger, J.M., Germond, J.F.: IEEE Trans. Med.
   Imaging **21**(12), 1504 (2002)
3. Burnett, S.S.C., Starkschall, G., Stevens, C.W., Liao, Z.: Med. Phys. **31**(2), 251 (2004)
4. Karangelis, G., Zimeras, S.: In: Meiler, M., Saupe, D., Kruggel, F., Handels, H., Lehmann, T.
   (eds.) Bildverarbeitung für die Medizin 2002, pp. 370–373. Springer, Berlin (2002)
5. Nyúl, L., Kanyó, J., Máté, E., Makay, G., Balogh, E., Fidrich, M., Kuba, A.: In: Gagalowicz, A.,
   Philips, W. (eds.) Computer Analysis of Images and Patterns, vol. 3691, pp. 456–463. Springer,
   Berlin (2005)
6. Kass, M., Witkin, A., Terzopoulos, D.: Int. J. Comput. Vis. **1**(4), 321 (1988)
7. Yao, J., O'Connor, S., Summers, R.: In: 3rd IEEE International Symposium on Biomedical
   Imaging: Nano to Macro, 2006, pp. 390–393 (2006)
8. Cremers, D., Rousson, M., Deriche, R.: Int. J. Comput. Vis. **72**(2), 195 (2007)
9. Grady, L.: IEEE Trans. Pattern Anal. Mach. Intell. **28**(11), 1768 (2006)
10. Wu, D., Liu, D., Puskas, Z., Lu, C., Wimmer, A., Tietjen, C., Soza, G., Zhou, S.: In: 2012 IEEE
    Conference on Computer Vision and Pattern Recognition (CVPR), pp. 980–987 (2012)
11. Tu, Z.: In: Tenth IEEE International Conference on Computer Vision, 2005. ICCV 2005, vol.
    2, pp. 1589–1596 (2005)
12. Andrews, S., Hamarneh, G., Saad, A.: In: Jiang, T., Navab, N., Pluim, J., Viergever, M. (eds.)
    Medical Image Computing and Computer-Assisted Intervention—MICCAI 2010, vol. 6363,
    pp. 9–16. Springer, Berlin (2010)

A Robust Segmentation Framework for Spine Trauma Diagnosis

Poay Hoon Lim, Ulas Bagci and Li Bai

Abstract Accurate three-dimensional (3D) image segmentation techniques have become increasingly important for medical image analysis in general, and for spinal vertebrae image analysis in particular. The complexity of vertebrae shapes, gaps in the cortical bone and internal boundaries pose significant challenge for image analysis. In this paper, we describe a level set image segmentation framework that integrates prior shape knowledge and local geometrical features to segment both normal and fractured spinal vertebrae. The prior shape knowledge is computed via kernel density estimation whereas the local geometrical features is captured through an edge-mounted Willmore energy. While the shape prior energy draws the level set function towards possible shape boundaries, the Willmore energy helps to capture the detail shape and curvature information of the vertebrae. Experiment on CT images of normal and fractured spinal vertebrae demonstrate promising results in 3D segmentation.

1 Introduction

Accurate 3D spinal vertebrae image segmentation techniques are important tools to assist the diagnosis and treatment of spinal disorders such as spine trauma [10, 14]. Severe spine injury can result in life threatening and chronological problems unless treated promptly and properly. In any spinal injury, the possibility of spinal frac-

P. H. Lim (✉) · L. Bai
School of Computer Science, University of Nottingham, Nottingham, UK
e-mail: psapl@nottingham.ac.uk

L. Bai
e-mail: bai@cs.nott.ac.uk

U. Bagci
Radiology and Imaging Sciences, National Institutes of Health, Bethesda, MD, USA
e-mail: ulas.bagci@nih.gov

J. Yao et al. (eds.), *Computational Methods and Clinical Applications*
for Spine Imaging, Lecture Notes in Computational Vision and Biomechanics 17,
DOI: 10.1007/978-3-319-07269-2_3, © Springer International Publishing Switzerland 2014

ture must be examined immediately. Image segmentation of spinal vertebrae in 3D allows detection, measurement, and monitoring of the fracture(s), and facilitates biomechanics analysis of the spinal column.

Despite an increasing interest in spinal vertebrae segmentation in recent years, accurate 3D segmentation methods for diseased or fractured vertebrae are still lacking. There are some existing works in the literature for 2D or 3D segmentations, however they often require user intervention or fall short in achieving high accuracy [4, 6–8, 11–13, 15]. Segmentation of diseased or fractured vertebrae has been attempted recently [5, 19, 20], however, these are either in 2D or focused only on vertebral body rather than the whole 3D spinal vertebrae.

Traumatic injury of the spine often correlates with morphometric features in images. Segmentation of the whole vertebra in 3D would facilitate the detection of fractured vertebra and the assessment of the severity of the fracture. For example, the highlighted volumetric region of vertebrae could assist physicians in performing visual inspection of vertebral fractures, determining its stability and measuring quantitatively the fractured vertebrae.

This work extends the spinal vertebrae segmentation method presented in [9] to segment fractured vertebrae. In this case, high variability of fractured vertebral shape is largely captured by the embedded Willmore flow, while prior shape energy comes into action only when encountering inhomogeneous image intensity distribution.

2 Segmentation Framework

It is well-known that level set methods have advantages such as flexibility in dealing with topological change, easy extension into higher dimensions, as well as easy integration of prior knowledge and region statistic. The segmentation framework presented here has made use of these properties. The framework combines the kernel density estimation technique and Willmore flow to incorporate prior shape knowledge and local geometrical features from images into the level set method. Whilst the prior shape model provides much needed prior knowledge when information is missing from the image, the edge-mounted Willmore flow helps to capture the local geometry and smoothes the evolving level set surface.

The level set method embeds an interface in a higher dimensional function ϕ (the signed distance function) as a level set $\phi = 0$ [16]. The evolution of the level set function $\phi(t)$ is governed by $\frac{\partial \phi}{\partial t} + F|\nabla \phi| = 0$, where F is the speed function. Based on the variational framework, an energy function $E(\phi)$ is defined in relation to the the speed function. The minimization of such energy generates the Euler-Lagrange equation, and the evolution of the equation is through calculus of variation:

$$\frac{\partial \phi}{\partial t} = -\frac{\partial E(\phi)}{\partial \phi}.$$

In this work, the fusion of energies whereby a shape prior distribution estimator E_s and an edge-mounted Willmore energy E_{w_0} is employed:

$$E(\phi) = \lambda E_s + E_{w_0},$$

where λ $(0 < \lambda \leq 1)$ is the weight parameter, which is tuned to suit the segmentation of normal and abnormal spinal vertebrae.

2.1 Computing Prior Shape Energy via Kernel Density Estimation

Kernel density estimation (KDE) is a nonparametric approach for estimating the probability density function of a random variable. Without assuming the prior shapes are Gaussian distributed, KDE presents advantage in estimating the shape distribution even with a small number of training set, in addition to modeling shapes with high complexity and structure. In this study, we adopted the prior shape energy formulation discussed by Cremers et al. [2].

The density estimation is formulated as a sum of Gaussian of shape dissimilarity measures $d^2(\phi, \phi_i)$, $i = 1, 2, \ldots, N$:

$$P(\phi) \propto \frac{1}{N} \sum_{i=1}^{N} e^{-\frac{d^2(\phi,\phi_i)}{2\sigma^2}},$$

where the shape dissimilarity measure $d^2(\phi, \phi_i)$ is defined as

$$d^2(\phi, \phi_i) = \int_\Omega \frac{1}{2} (H(\phi) - H(\phi_m))^2 \, dx,$$

$$\sigma^2 = \frac{1}{N} \sum_{i=1}^{N} \min_{j \neq i} d^2(\phi_i, \phi_j),$$

and $H(\phi)$ is the *Heaviside* function. By maximizing the conditional probability

$$P(\phi|I) = \frac{P(I|\phi)P(\phi)}{P(I)},$$

and considering the shape energy as

$$E_s(\phi) = -\log P(\phi|I),$$

the variational with respect to ϕ becomes

$$\frac{\partial E_s}{\partial \phi} = \frac{\sum_{i=1}^{N} \alpha_i \frac{\partial}{\partial \phi} d^2(\phi, \phi_i)}{2\sigma^2 \sum_{i=1}^{N} \alpha_i}$$

$$= \sum_{i=1}^{N} \frac{e^{-\frac{d^2(\phi, \phi_i)}{2\sigma^2}}}{2\sigma^2 \sum_{i=1}^{N} \alpha_i} \left(2\delta(\phi) \left[H(\phi) - H(\phi_i(x - \mu_\phi)) \right] \right.$$

$$\left. + \int \left[H(\phi(\xi)) - H(\phi_i(\xi - \mu_\phi)) \right] \delta\phi(\xi) \frac{(x - \mu_\phi)^T \nabla\phi(\xi)}{\int H\phi dx} d\xi \right),$$

where μ_ϕ is the centroid of ϕ and $\alpha_i = \exp\left(-\frac{1}{2\sigma^2} d^2(\phi, \phi_i)\right)$ is the weight factor for $i = 1, 2, \ldots, N$.

2.2 Computing Local Geometry Energy via Willmore Flow

Willmore energy is a function of mean curvature, which is a quantitative measure of how much a given surface deviates from a sphere. It is formulated as

$$E_w = \frac{1}{2} \int_M h^2 dA,$$

where M is a d-dimensional surface embedded in $\mathbb{R}^{d+1}$ and h the mean curvature on M [18]. For image segmentation, the Willmore energy provides an internal energy that gives a useful description of a region, where the effect of edge indicator is not significant. In these regions, smoothness of the shape of the curve should be maintained and extended, which can be regarded as a weak form of inpainting [3].

As a geometric functional, the Willmore energy is defined on the geometric representation of a collection of level sets. Its gradient flow can be well represented by defining a suitable metric, the Frobenius norm, on the space of the level sets. Frobenius norm is a convenient choice as it is equivalent to the l^2-norm of a matrix and more importantly it is computationally attainable. As Frobenius norm is an inner-product norm, the optimization in the variational method comes naturally.

Based on the formulation by Droske and Rumpf [3], the Willmore flow or the variational form for the Willmore energy with respect to ϕ is

$$\frac{\partial E_w}{\partial \phi} = -\|\nabla\phi\| \left(\Delta_M h + h(t) \left(\|S(t)\|_2^2 - \frac{1}{2} h(t)^2 \right) \right),$$

where $\Delta_M h = \Delta h - h \frac{\partial h}{\partial n} - \frac{\partial^2 h}{\partial n^2}$ is the Laplacian Beltrami operator on h with $n = \frac{\nabla\phi}{\|\nabla\phi\|}$, $S = (I - n \otimes n)(\nabla \times \nabla)\phi$ is the shape operator on ϕ and $\|S\|_2$ is the Frobenius norm of S.

Table 1 Average DSC (%) and HD (mm) with standard deviation for segmentations of normal lumbar vertebrae (L1 to L5) using Chan-Vese (CV), Chan-Vese with prior shape (CV + S), Caselles (Ca), Caselles with prior shape (Ca + S), edge-mounted Willmore (W_0), edge-mounted Willmore with prior shape (W_0 + S) energies, region growing (RG) and graph cut (GC) approach

Method	DSC (%)	HD (mm)
CV	37.68 ± 7.07	26.68 ± 2.18
CVS	45.09 ± 7.54	25.31 ± 2.38
Ca	55.75 ± 8.14	22.22 ± 1.57
CaS	71.12 ± 2.72	18.39 ± 1.15
W	75.82 ± 2.81	19.21 ± 1.51
WS	**89.32±1.70**	**14.30 ± 1.40**
RG	42.30 ± 11.43	25.20 ± 2.30
GC	13.23 ± 11.11	63.22 ± 14.82

In order to ensure the smoothing effect work successfully around the constructed surface and not affecting the desired edge of vertebrae, the Willmore flow is coupled with the edge indicator function $g(I) = \frac{1}{1+|\nabla G_\sigma * I|^2}$, where G_σ is the Gaussian filter with standard deviation σ:

$$\frac{\partial E_{w_0}}{\partial \phi} = g(I)\frac{\partial E_w}{\partial \phi}.$$

3 Experiments and Results

Experiments have been conducted on CT images of spinal vertebrae for 2D and 3D segmentation. The dataset consists of 20 CT images of normal and 4 CT images of fractured spinal vertebrae images of patients aged 18 to 66 years. The images were acquired from various CT scanners such as a 32-detector row Siemens definition, 64-detector row Philips Brilliance and 320-detector row Toshiba Aquilion. The in plane resolutions for these sagittal images range from 0.88 to 1.14 mm, with consistent slice thickness of 2 mm. Original images for these images have fixed sizes of 512 × 512, with number of slices varying from 45 to 98. For 3D segmentation, a torus is set manually surrounding the spinal canal as the initial contour. The level set method is then implemented using a narrow band scheme [1] with a re-initialization algorithm [17].

It has been reported that the 3D segmentations of spinal vertebrae clearly outperform the other methods such as region growing, graph cut, the classical level set methods such as Chan-Vese and Caselles models as well as their combinations with shape priors [9]. While some methods can perform relatively well in the 2D segmentation of spinal vertebrae, the majority of them fail badly when extended to the 3D segmentation of an individual vertebra due to the highly complex shape and connected structure as well as the nonuniform image intensity distribution in the pos-

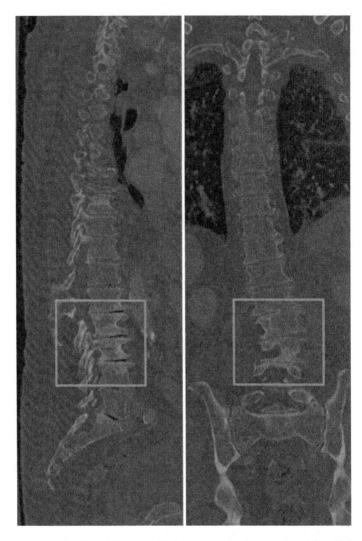

Fig. 1 An example of patient CT image with fractures on lumbar vertebrae L2 and L3

terior column of vertebra. Table 1 summarized 3D segmentation results on normal lumbar vertebrae using various approach, evaluated with ground truth. It is worth noted the effectiveness of our segmentation framework, with an overall accuracy of $89.32 \pm 1.70\,\%$ and 14.03 ± 1.40 mm based on Dice similarity coefficient and Hausdorff distance respectively, whilst the inter- and intra-observer variation agreements were $92.11 \pm 1.97\,\%$, $94.94 \pm 1.69\,\%$, 3.32 ± 0.46 mm and 3.80 ± 0.56 mm. Segmentation results depend highly on available dataset. The intra- and inter-observer variation estimations were performed to verify the difficulty of manual delineation in 3D using our dataset. We have shown that our results present no significant sta-

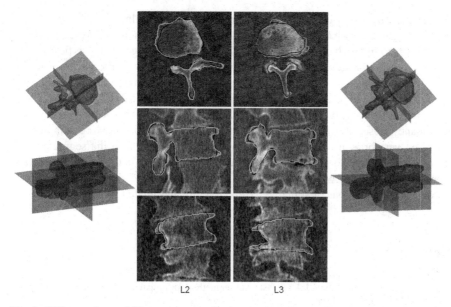

Fig. 2 Different views of 3D segmentation for fractured lumbar vertebrae L2 and L3 as well as their projections in 2D (*red*) compared with manual segmentation (*yellow*) on axial, sagittal and coronal views

tistical differences ($p > 0.05$) when compared with these observer estimations. The robustness of the proposed segmentation framework is demonstrated on the CT image of a patient with fractures on lumbar vertebrae L2 and L3 as seen in Fig. 1. As shown in Fig. 2, the segmentation framework manages to capture the 3D shape of fractured vertebrae L2 and L3, despite the inhomogeneity, noise and missing edges appeared on these fractured vertebra images. It enables individual segmentation of vertebrae without leaking into the nearby connected vertebra. Segmentation results on fractured vertebrae were evaluated via visual inspection by radiologist.

4 Discussion and Conclusion

An accurate level set segmentation framework for segmenting spinal vertebrae in 2D and 3D is presented in this study. The robustness of the framework is demonstrated on CT images of fractured vertebrae. The framework combines the kernel density estimation technique and Willmore flow to incorporate prior shape knowledge and local geometrical features from images into the level set method. It is worth noted that fusion of these energies effectively translate the prior shape knowledge and local geometrical feature of spinal vertebrae into the level set segmentation framework. The Willmore flow driven level set segmentation demonstrates better regularization than the widely used mean curvature flow in level set segmentation. Unlike minimizing surface area by mean curvature flow in regularization, Willmore flow minimizes the bending energy when performing surface smoothing, which is more suitable for object with complex shape and structure. The segmentation algorithm was performed directly in a 3D volumetric manner instead of sequentially to the slices of a 3D image. This allows the volumetric tissue connectivity be taken into consideration and hence, enables more meaningful representation of 3D anatomical shape and structure. Moreover, it forms a continuous, smooth 3D surface and without the post processing redundancy posed by the slice by slice segmentation approach. More samples of fractured vertebrae are needed to perform further evaluation on the segmentation framework. Future work will integrate the algorithm into a pathological vertebrae characterization framework to yield an efficient computer aided diagnosis platform for quantitative analysis of spinal vertebrae fracture and related problems.

References

1. Adalsteinsson, D., Sethian, J.A.: A fast level set method for propagating interfaces. J. Comput. Phys. **118**, 269–277 (1995)
2. Cremers, D., Osher, S.J., Soatto, S.: Kernel density estimation and intrinsic alignment for shape priors in level set segmentation. Int. J. Comput. Vis. **69**(3), 335–351 (2006)
3. Droske, M., Rumpf, M.: A level set formulation for willmore flow. Interfaces Free Boundaries **6**(3), 361–378 (2004)
4. Ghebreab, S., Smeulders, A.: Combining strings and necklaces for interactive three-dimensional segmentation of spinal images using an integral deformable spine model. IEEE Trans. Biomed. Eng. **51**(10), 1821–1829 (2004)
5. Ghosh, S., Raja's, A., Chaudhary, V, Dhillon, G.: Automatic lumbar vertebra segmentation from clinical CT for wedge compression fracture diagnosis. In: SPIE Medical, Imaging (2011)
6. Kadoury, S., Labelle, H., Pargios, N.: Automatic inference of articulated spine models in CT images using higher-order markov random fields. Medical Image Analysis **15**, 426–437 (2011)
7. Kang, Y., Engelke, K., Kalender, W.A.: A new accurate and precise 3d segmentation method for skeletal structures in volumetric ct data. IEEE Trans. Med. Imag. **22**(5), 586–598 (2003)
8. Klinder, T., Ostermann, J., Ehm, M., Franz, A., Kneser, R., Lorenz, C.: Automated model-based vertebra detection, identification, and segmentation in ct images. Med. Image Anal. **13**(3), 471–482 (2009)
9. Lim, P., Bagci, U., Bai, L.: Introducing willmore flow into level set segmentation of spinal vertebrae. IEEE Trans. Biomed. Eng. **60**(1), 115–122 (2013)
10. Looby, S., Flanders, A.: Spine trauma. Radiol. Clin. N. Am. **49**(1), 129–163 (2011)
11. Lorenz, C., Krahnstoever, N.: 3D statistical shape models for medical image segmentation. In: 3D Digital Imaging and Modeling, pp. 4–8 (1999)
12. Ma, J., Lu, L., Zhan, Y., Zhou, X., Salganicoff, M., Krishnan, A.: Hierarchical segmentation and identification of thoracic vertebra using learning-based edge detection and coarse-to-fine deformable model. In: MICCAI, pp. 19–27 (2010)
13. Mastmeyer, A., Engelke, K., Fuchs, C., Kalender, W.A.: A hierarchical 3-d segmentation method and the definition of vertebral body coordinate systems for qct of the lumbar spine. Med. Image Anal. **10**, 560–577 (2006)
14. Mayer, M., Zenner, J., Auffarth, A., Blocher, M., Figl, M., Resch, H., Koller, H.: Hidden discoligamentous instability in cervical spine injuries: can quantitative motion analysis improve detection? Eur. Spine J. **22**(10), 2219–2227 (2013)
15. Naegel, B.: Using mathematical morphology for the anatomical labeling of vertebrae from 3-d ct-scan images. Comput. Med. Imag. Grap. **31**(3), 141–156 (2007)

16. Osher, S., Sethian, J.: Fronts propagating with curvature-dependent speed: algorithms based on hamilton-jacobi formulations. J. Comput. Phys. **79**, 12–49 (1988)
17. Sussman, M., Smereka, P., Osher, S.: A level set approach for computing solutions to incompressible 2-phase flow. J. Comput. Phys. **114**(1), 146–159 (1994)
18. Willmore, T.J.: Note on embedded surfaces. Analele Ştiinţifice ale Universităţii Al. I. Cuza din Iaşi. Serie Nouă Ia **11B**, 493–496 (1965)
19. Yao, J., Burns, J.E., Munoz, H., Summers, R.M.: Detection of vertebral body fractures based on cortical shell unwrapping. In: MICCAI Part III, LNCS 7512 (2012)
20. Yao, J., Burns, J.E., Wiese, T., Summers, R.M.: Quantitative vertebral compression fracture evaluation using a height compass. In: SPIE Medical Imaging (2012)

2D-PCA Based Tensor Level Set Framework for Vertebral Body Segmentation

Ahmed Shalaby, Aly Farag and Melih Aslan

Abstract In this paper, a novel statistical shape modeling method is developed for the vertebral body (VB) segmentation framework. Two-dimensional principal component analysis (2D-PCA) technique is exploited to extract the shape prior. The obtained shape model is then embedded into the image domain to develop a new shape-based segmentation approach. Our framework consists of four main steps: (1) shape model construction using 2D-PCA, (2) the detection of the VB region using the Matched filter, (3) initial segmentation using a new region-based tensor level set model, and (4) registration of the shape priors and initially segmented region to obtain the final segmentation. The proposed method is validated on a Phantom as well as clinical CT images with various Gaussian noise levels. The experimental results show that the noise immunity and the segmentation accuracy of our framework are much higher than scalar level sets approaches. Additionally, the construction of the shape model using 2D-PCA is computationally more efficient than PCA.

1 Introduction

The vertebra consists of the vertebral body (VB), spinous (spinal) processes, pedicles, and other anatomical regions (see Fig. 1). Spinous processes, pedicles, and ribs should not be included in the bone mineral density (BMD) measurements since the BMD measurements are restricted to the VBs. The VB segmentation is not an easy task since

A. Shalaby (✉) · A. Farag · M. Aslan
Computer Vision and Image Processing Laboratory, University of Louisville,
Louisville, KY, USA
e-mail: ahmed.shalaby@louisville.edu

A. Farag
e-mail: aly.farag@louisville.edu

M. Aslan
e-mail: melih.aslan@louisville.edu

J. Yao et al. (eds.), *Computational Methods and Clinical Applications*
for Spine Imaging, Lecture Notes in Computational Vision and Biomechanics 17,
DOI: 10.1007/978-3-319-07269-2_4, © Springer International Publishing Switzerland 2014

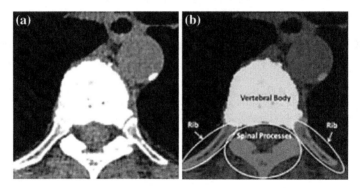

Fig. 1 The region of interest in our experiment: **a** A clinical CT slice of a human vertebra. **b** The *blue color* shows the VB region

the ribs and spinal processes have similar gray level information. There are limited publications for vertebrae segmentation. For instance, Kang et al. [11] proposed a 3D segmentation method for skeletal structures from CT data. Their method is a multi-step method that starts with a three dimensional region growing step using local adaptive thresholds, followed by a closing of boundary discontinuities and then an anatomically-oriented boundary adjustment. Mastmeyer et al. [12] presented a hierarchical segmentation approach only for the lumbar spine in order to measure the bone mineral density. The detection of the vertebrae is carried out manually. The authors reported that complete analysis of three vertebrae took 10 min in 2006 on a "high standard PC system". This timing is far from the real time required for clinical applications but it is a huge improvement compared to the timing of 1–2 h reported in [10]. Aslan et al. proposed various methods to segment VBs in [2–5, 7] which can be considered as progressive VB segmentation studies. In [5], the shape model was not used and it was assumed that the detection rate of VBs was very accurate for cropping the pedicles automatically. In [3], a probabilistic shape model was introduced in addition to the intensity and spatial interaction information to enhance the results. However, the shape model was assumed to be registered to the object of interest manually. In [2, 4, 7], the probabilistic shape model was automatically embedded into image domain and they appeared to be more realistic experiments. In [7], the scalar level sets model which needs manual initialization was used, and was validated on a limited number of data sets. In [2], the shape prior is extracted using PCA on signed distance functions (SDF) of all training images. Then shape model was registered into the image domain using the gradient descent approach [1]. In this paper, a region-based tensor level set model is initially used for segmenting the input CT image. This model introduces a three-order tensor to comprehensively depict features of pixels, e.g., gray value and the local geometrical features, such as orientation and gradient [14]. Additionally, we excerpt the shape model construction method described in [13]. This method adopts the 2D-PCA approach to build the shape prior instead of conventional PCA [15]. The rest of the paper is organized

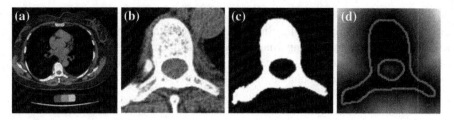

Fig. 2 An example of the initial labeling. **a** Original CT image, **b** detection of the VB region using MF, **c** the initial labeling, f* using tensor level set segmentation and **d** the SDF of the initial segmentation (f*) which is used in the registration phase. *Red color* shows the zero level contour

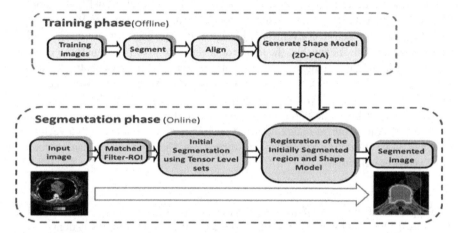

Fig. 3 Our proposed shape-based segmentation. Our framework consists of two main stages; the training phase and the segmentation phase

as follows: Sect. 2 discusses the background of methods used in our experiment. Section 3 explains the experiments, and compares our results with other alternatives. Finally, conclusions are drawn in Sect. 4.

2 Methods

Intensity based model may not be enough to obtain the optimum segmentation. Hence, we propose a new shape based segmentation method. This method has several steps. As a pre-processing step, we extract the human spine area using the Matched filter (MF) adopted in [6]. As shown in Fig. 2a, b, the MF is employed to detect the VB automatically. This process helps to roughly remove the spinous processes and pedicles. Additionally, it eliminates the user interaction. We tested the Matched filter using 3,000 clinical CT images. The VB detection accuracy is 97.6 %. In the second phase, we obtain initial labeling (f*) using the region-based tensor level set model, as described in [14]. Finally, we register the initial labeled image and the shape priors to obtain the optimum labeling, as in [1]. To obtain the shape priors (p), we use the 2D-PCA on all training images. Figure 3 summarizes the main components of our framework. The following sections give more details about the shape model construction and the segmentation method.

2.1 Shape Model Construction

In this work, we describe the shape representation using the SDF, as in [2]. The objective of this step is to obtain the most important information of training images using 2D-PCA. As op-posed to conventional PCA, 2D-PCA is based on 2D matrix rather than 1D vector. This means that, the image does not need to be pre-transformed into a vector. In addition, the image covariance matrix(G) can be directly constructed using the original image matrices. As a result, 2D-PCA has two important advantages over PCA. First, it is easier to evaluate G accurately since its size using 2D-PCA is much smaller. Second, less time is required to determine the corresponding eigenvectors [15]. 2D-PCA projects an image matrix X, which is an mn matrix onto a vector, b, which is an n1 vector, by the linear transformation. The resultant projection coefficient vector y will be:

$$\mathbf{y}=\mathbf{X}b. \tag{1}$$

Suppose that there are M training images, the ith training image is denoted by $\mathbf{X}_i$, $(i = 1, 2, \ldots, M)$ and the average image of all training samples is denoted by $\overline{\mathbf{X}}=\frac{1}{M}\sum_{i=1}^{M}\mathbf{X}_i$. Then, let us define the image covariance matrix $\mathbf{G}$, as in [15]:

$$\mathbf{G}=\frac{1}{M}\sum_{i=1}^{M}(\mathbf{X}_i-\overline{\mathbf{X}})^t\,(\mathbf{X}_i-\overline{\mathbf{X}})\,. \tag{2}$$

It is clear that, the matrix $\mathbf{G}$ is $n \times n$ nonnegative definite matrix. Similar to PCA, the goal of 2D-PCA is to find a projection axis that maximizes $\mathbf{b}^t\mathbf{G}b$. The optimal K projection axes $\mathbf{b}_k$, where $k = 1, 2, \ldots, K$, that maximize the above criterion are the eigenvectors of $\mathbf{G}$ corresponding to the largest K eigenvalues. For an image $\mathbf{X}$, we can use its reconstruction $\widetilde{\mathbf{X}}$ defined below to approximate it.

$$\widetilde{\mathbf{X}} = \overline{\mathbf{X}} + \int_{k=1}^{K} \mathbf{y}_k\mathbf{b_k}^t, \tag{3}$$

where $\mathbf{y}_k = (\mathbf{X}-\overline{\mathbf{X}})\,\mathbf{b_k}$ is called the kth principal component vector of the sample image $\mathbf{X}$. The principal component vectors obtained are used to form an $m \times K$ matrix $\mathbf{Y} = [\mathbf{y}_1,\mathbf{y}_2,\ldots,\mathbf{y}_K]$ and let $\mathbf{B} = [\mathbf{b}_1,\mathbf{b}_2,\ldots,\mathbf{b}_K]$, then we can rewrite Eq. 3 as:

$$\widetilde{\mathbf{X}} = \overline{\mathbf{X}} + \mathbf{Y}\mathbf{B}^t. \tag{4}$$

However, one disadvantage of 2D-PCA (compared to PCA) is that more coefficients are needed to represent an image. From Eq. 4, it is clear that dimension of the 2D-PCA principal component matrix $\mathbf{Y}$ ($m \times K$) is always much higher than PCA. To reduce the dimension of matrix $\mathbf{Y}$, the conventional PCA is used for further dimensional reduction after 2D-PCA. More details will be discussed in the following section.

Now, let the training set consists of M training images $\{I_1,..., I_M\}$; with SDFs $\{\Phi_1, ..., \Phi_M\}$. All images are binary, pre-aligned, and normalized to the same resolution. As in [2], we obtain the mean level set function of the training shapes, $\overline{\Phi}$, as the average of these M signed distance functions. To extract the shape variabilities, $\overline{\Phi}$ is subtracted from each of the training SDFs. The obtained mean-offset functions can be represented as $\{\widehat{\Phi}_1, ..., \widehat{\Phi}_M\}$. These new functions are used to measure the variabilities of the training images. We use 80 training VB images with 120×120 pixels in our experiment. According (2), the constructed matrix $\mathbf{G}$ will be:

$$\mathbf{G} = \frac{1}{M} \sum_{i=1}^{M=80} \widehat{\Phi}_i^t \widehat{\Phi}_i. \tag{5}$$

Experimentally, we find that, the minimum suitable value is $K = 10$. Less than this value, the accuracy of our segmentation algorithm falls drastically. After choosing the eigenvectors corresponding to 10 largest eigenvalues, $\mathbf{b}_1, \mathbf{b}_2, ..., \mathbf{b}_{10}$, we obtained the principal component matrix $\mathbf{Y}_i$($m = 120 \times K = 10$) for each SDF of our training set ($i = 1, 2, ..., 80$). For more dimensional reduction, the conventional PCA is applied on the principal components $\{\overrightarrow{\mathbf{Y}}_1,..., \overrightarrow{\mathbf{Y}}_\mathbf{M}\}$. It should be noted that, $\overrightarrow{\mathbf{Y}}$ is the vector representation of $\mathbf{Y}$. The reconstructed components (after retransforming to matrix representation) will be:

$$\widetilde{\mathbf{Y}}_{\{l,h\}} = \mathbf{U}\mathbf{e}_{\{l,h\}}, \tag{6}$$

where $\mathbf{U}$ is the matrix which contains L eigenvectors corresponding to L largest eigenvalues λ_l, ($l = 1, 2, ..., L$), and $\mathbf{e}_{\{l,h\}}$ is the set of model parameters which can be described as

$$\mathbf{e}_{\{l,h\}} = h\sqrt{\lambda_l}, \tag{7}$$

where $l = 1, ..., L$, $h = \{-, ..., \}$, and is a constant which can be chosen arbitrarily (in our experiments, we chose $L = 4, = 3$). The new principal components of training SDFs are represented as $\{\widetilde{\mathbf{Y}}_1,..., \widetilde{\mathbf{Y}}_\mathbf{N}\}$ instead of $\{\mathbf{Y}_1,..., \mathbf{Y}_\mathbf{M}\}$ where N is the multiplication of L and standard deviation in eigenvalues (the number of elements in h), i.e. $N = L(2 + 1)$. Given the set $\{\widetilde{\mathbf{Y}}_1,..., \widetilde{\mathbf{Y}}_\mathbf{N}\}$, the new projected training SDFs are obtained as follows:

$$\widetilde{\Phi}_j = \overline{\Phi} + \widetilde{\mathbf{Y}}_j \mathbf{B}^t, \quad j = 1, 2, ..., N. \tag{8}$$

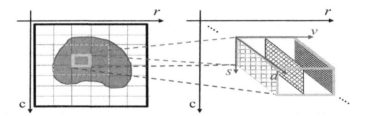

Fig. 4 The tensor representation for each pixel in an image

Finally, the shape model is required to capture the variations in the training set. This model is considered to be a weighted sum of the projected SDFs (Eq. 8) as follows:

$$\Phi_{\mathbf{p}} = \sum_{j=1}^{N} w_j \widetilde{\Phi}_j. \tag{9}$$

Let $\mathbf{w} = [w_1, \ldots, w_N]^t$ to be the weighting coefficient vector. By varying these weights, $\Phi_{\mathbf{p}}$ can cover all values of the training distance functions and, hence, the shape model changes according to all of the given images [13].

2.2 Segmentation Method

To estimate the initial labeling $\mathbf{f}^*$, we use the tensor level set method described in [14]. An example of the initial labeling is shown in Fig. 2c. To segment an image more accurately, more overall information in the image to be segmented should be considered by the segmentation algorithms, and more suitable representation for the information should be used to depict the image. As in [14], we build a tensor representation for a pixel. This tensor representation contains more information (e.g., average gray value, gradient, and orientation) and is relatively overall. As illustrated in Fig. 4, the construction of the unified tensor representation contains three steps:

1. To make our model more robust against noise, the initial image is smoothed by a Gaussian filter bank, and then, the gray value of each pixel in the smoothed image is included into the unified tensor representation as a matrix written as:

$$[T_{r,c}^{s,d,v=1}]_{S \times D} = \frac{1}{\sqrt{SD}} \begin{bmatrix} G_{\sigma 1}(u_{r,c}) & \cdots & G_{\sigma 1}(u_{r,c}) \\ \vdots & \ddots & \vdots \\ G_{\sigma_s}(u_{r,c}) & \cdots & G_{\sigma_s}(u_{r,c}) \end{bmatrix}_{S \times D} \tag{10}$$

where $T_{r,c}^{s,d,v=1}$ is an element in the three-order tensor representation. s denotes the scale, and its maximum number is S. d is the direction, and its maximum number is D (where $S = 4$ and $D = 8$ as in [14]). $u_{r,c}$ is the image to be segmented, and $G_{\sigma 1,...,\sigma_s}(.)$ is the output generated by using the Gaussian function having different standard deviations convolving with the image.

2. The gray value of each pixel in the image to be segmented is embed into the unified tensor representation, and the process is formulated as:

$$[T_{r,c}^{s,d,v=2}]_{S \times D} = \frac{1}{\sqrt{SD}} [u_{r,c}]_{S \times D} \tag{11}$$

3. The Gabor features are used to represent the gradient and orientation of images. Having the Gabor functions defined by [14] convolved with the image to be segmented, the Gabor-based image representation in $R^{m \times n \times 4 \times 8}$ is obtained. Thus, a rule of correspondence between a pixel of the image and a matrix in $R^{4 \times 8}$ is built as follows:

$$[T_{r,c}^{s,d,v=3}]_{S \times D} = [Gabor\ (u_{r,c})]_{S \times D} \tag{12}$$

where $Gabor()$ is the outputs generated by convolving the Gabor functions with the image [14].

Therefore, an image is projected on a five-order tensor in $R^{m \times n \times 4 \times 8 \times 3}$. The first two indexes give the pixel location, and the last three indexes give the three-order tensor representation.

Now, assume that we have an evolving curve C in $\Omega \in R^{m \times n \times}$ that divides the field T into two regions, i.e., $\omega \in R^{m \times n \times}$, $\omega^c \in R^{m \times n \times}$, and $C = \partial \omega$. Then, we assume that the field T is composed of these two homogenous regions and further assume that the object to be detected in the field is with the similar value. The fitting error between this piecewise constant representation and the field T is E_e. Adding a regularizing term E_g, the energy functional is defined as

$$E\ (C) =\ E_g + E_e \tag{13}$$

E_g denotes the geometrical feature of the evolving curve, i.e., the length of the curve. Accompanied with the decreasing of this energy, the fitting term is minimized, and the segmentation result is obtained. According to [14], the energy functional will be:

$$E\left(\Phi, c_+^{s,d,v}, c_-^{s,d,v}\right) = \zeta \int_\Omega \delta(\Phi)|\nabla \Phi|d\Omega + \varepsilon_+ \int_\Omega dist_\Omega^2\left(T_\Omega^{s,d,v}, c_+^{s,d,v}\right) H(\Phi)d\Omega$$

$$+ \varepsilon_- \int_\Omega dist_\Omega^2\left(T_\Omega^{s,d,v}, c_-^{s,d,v}\right)(1 - H\ (\Phi))d\Omega \tag{14}$$

where $c_+^{s,d,v}$, $c_-^{s,d,v}$ are the averages in tensor form of the regions inside and outside the evolving curve C, respectively, ζ is the weight of the regularizing term. ε_+ and ε_- are the weights of the fitting term, $H()$ is the Heaviside step function, and $\delta()$ is the Dirac delta function. We use the same method described in [14] to minimize this energy functional based on Euler–Lagrange equation for the unknown level set function Φ. More details about the numerical solution can be found in [14]. As a result of this optimization process, the initially segmented region is acquired and is then used to obtain the SDF (Φ_{f*}). To use the shape prior in the segmentation process, we need to register $\mathbf{f}^*$ and the shape prior $\mathbf{p}$. The objective of the shape registration problem is to find the point-wise transformation between any two given shapes α and β minimizing a certain energy function based on some dissimilarity measure. In this paper, we follow the similar notation scheme in [2]. Let us define the result by β that is obtained by applying a transformation $\mathbf{A}$ (with scale, rotation, and translation parameters) to a given contour/surface α (It is clear that β and α correspond to $\mathbf{f}^*$ and $\mathbf{p}$). The shape representation used in this work changes the problem from the 2D/3D shape to the higher dimensional representation. Hence, we will look for a transformation $\mathbf{A}$ that gives pixel-wise correspondences between the two shape representations Φ_α and Φ_β.

For the 2D case, we assume that the transformation has scaling components, $\mathbf{S} = \begin{bmatrix} s_x & 0 \\ 0 & s_y \end{bmatrix}$, rotation angles $\mathbf{R} = \begin{bmatrix} \cos(\theta) & -\sin(\theta) \\ \sin(\theta) & \cos(\theta) \end{bmatrix}$, and translations represented as $\mathbf{Tr} = \begin{bmatrix} t_x & t_y \end{bmatrix}^t$. So, the transformation will be in the form $\mathbf{A(X)} = \mathbf{SRX} + \mathbf{Tr}$. After scaling the components of the Φ_{f*} by $\mathbf{A}$, the dissimilarity measure will be:

$$\mathbf{r} = \mathbf{SR}\Phi_p - \Phi_{f*}(\mathbf{A}) \tag{15}$$

and the squared magnitude of the above measure is summed over the image domain Ω to get an optimization energy function:

$$E\left(\Phi_\mathbf{p}, \Phi_{\mathbf{f}*}\right) = \int_\Omega \delta_\varepsilon\left(\Phi_\mathbf{p}, \Phi_{\mathbf{f}*}\right) \mathbf{r}^T \mathbf{r} d\Omega , \tag{16}$$

where δ_ε is an indicator function defined as:

$$\delta_\varepsilon(\Phi_\mathbf{p}, \Phi_{\mathbf{f}*}) = \begin{cases} 0 & if\,min\left(|\Phi_\mathbf{p}|, |\Phi_{\mathbf{f}*}|\right) > \varepsilon \\ 1 & if\,min\left(|\Phi_\mathbf{p}|, |\Phi_{\mathbf{f}*}|\right) \le \varepsilon \end{cases} , \tag{17}$$

Due to δ_ε, all pixels of a distance (measured from the nearest point on the boundary) greater than ε are not considered in the energy optimization problem which reduces the computational time of our problem (Narrow-banding effect). As in [13], after applying the gradient descent method, it is clear that:

$$\frac{d}{dt}s_\mathbf{i} = 2\int_\Omega \delta_\varepsilon(\Phi_\mathbf{p}, \Phi_{\mathbf{f}*})\mathbf{r}^T[\nabla_{s_i}\mathbf{S}\Phi_\mathbf{p} - \nabla\Phi_{\mathbf{f}*}^T\nabla_{s_i}\mathbf{A}]d\Omega,$$

$$\frac{d}{dt}\theta_\mathbf{i} = 2\int_\Omega \delta_\varepsilon\left(\Phi_\mathbf{p}, \Phi_{\mathbf{f}*}\right)\mathbf{r}^T\left[\nabla\Phi_\mathbf{p}^T\nabla_{\theta_i}\mathbf{A}\right]d\Omega,$$

$$\frac{d}{dt} t_{\mathbf{i}} = 2 \int_{\Omega} \delta_{\varepsilon} \left(\Phi_{\mathbf{p}}, \Phi_{\mathbf{f}*} \right) \mathbf{r}^{T} \left[\nabla \Phi_{\mathbf{f}*}^{T} \nabla_{t_i} \mathbf{A} \right] d\Omega, \tag{18}$$

where $s_i \in \{s_x, s_y\}$, $\theta_i \in \{\theta_x, \theta_y\}$ and $t_i \in \{T_x, T_y\}$ of the transformation $\mathbf{A}$. Regarding to the weighting coefficients w_n's (9), and similar to [1], the energy function is a quadratic function of this weights, which leads to a closed-form when the derivatives with respect to the weights are zeros:

$$\Psi \mathbf{w} = \Lambda \tag{19}$$

where Λ is a column vector of size N and Ψ is and $N \times N$ matrix. Their elements are calculated as follows:

$$\Lambda_{\mathbf{i}} = \int_{\Omega} \delta_{\varepsilon}(\Phi_{\mathbf{p}}, \Phi_{\mathbf{f}*})[\mathbf{S}\Phi_{\mathbf{f}*} - \overline{\Phi}(\mathbf{A})]^{T} [\widetilde{\Phi}_i(\mathbf{A}) - \overline{\Phi}(\mathbf{A})] d\Omega, \tag{20}$$

$$\Psi_{\mathbf{i}j} = \int_{\Omega} \delta_{\varepsilon}(\Phi_{\mathbf{p}}, \Phi_{\mathbf{f}*}))[\widetilde{\Phi}_j(\mathbf{A}) - \overline{\Phi}(\mathbf{A})]^{T} [\widetilde{\Phi}_i(\mathbf{A}) - \overline{\Phi}(\mathbf{A})] d\Omega, \tag{21}$$

$\forall (i, j) \in [1, N] \times [1, N]$. Using unique training shapes (with variabilities not identical) guarantees that Ψ is a positive definite matrix avoiding singularity.

3 Experimental Results

In this paper, we apply the proposed framework on clinical CT spine bone images. The clinical datasets were scanned at 120 kV and 3.0, 2.5, 1.33 mm, or 0.67 mm slice thickness. We tested our algorithm on 1400 CT slices/72 VBs which are obtained from 22 different patients. The goal is to segment the VB region correctly. The segmentation accuracy and robustness of our framework are tested on the phantom named as the European Spine Phantom (ESP) as well as the clinical datasets. All algorithms are implemented using Matlab 7.[1]

To assess the proposed method under various challenges, we added a zero mean Gaussian noise with different signal-to-noise ratios (SNR)—from 0 to 100 dB—to our CT images. The segmentation accuracy is measured for each method using the ground truths. It should be noted that the ground truths are manually segmented and then validated by a radiologist. We calculate the percentage segmentation accuracy (Acc) using Dice coefficient as follows:

$$Acc\% = 100 \times (\frac{2TP}{FP + 2TP + FN}), \tag{22}$$

---

[1] All algorithms are run on a PC with a 2 Ghz Core i7 Quad processor with 6 GB RAM.

Fig. 5 Definitions of the accuracy terminologies

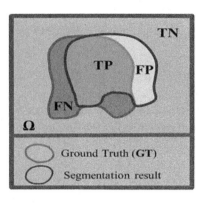

where FP represents the false positive (i.e. the total number of the misclassified pixels of the background), FN is the false negative (i.e. the total number of the misclassified pixels of the object), and TP is the true positive (i.e. total number of the correctly classified pixels). See Fig. 5.

We used a variety of methods to measure the accuracy of our framework. First, we used the visual inspection to evaluate the segmentation quality of our approach. Figure 6 compares the results of different examples for the initial segmentation step using the scalar level sets method [8] and the tensor level set model [14] which is used in our proposed framework. As shown in this figure, the scalar level sets method fails to segment the whole vertebra in many cases. However, the tensor level sets approach can segment them well. Additionally, the boundaries detected by scalar level sets are not smooth, and some obvious boundaries are not detected. The tensor level sets method segments the image accurately. Figure 7 shows various segmentation results of three different methods applied on some clinical datasets. These methods are: (i) The PCA based segmentation described in [2] (but using the tensor level set as initial labeling instead of graph cuts), and (2) Our 2D-PCA based tensor level segmentation. The segmentation accuracies of the 2D-PCA based results shown in row (ii) are: 94.3, and 91.2 % respectively. For PCA based results in row (i), the segmentation accuracies are: 86.2, and 84.9 % respectively. It is clear that our method is more accurate than the method in [2]. Figure 8 studies the effect of the initialization on our proposed framework. Results indicate that the performance of our method is almost constant with different initialization parameters. To quantitatively demonstrate the accuracy of our approach, we calculate the average segmentation accuracy of our segmentation method on 1400 CT images under various signal-to-noise ratios and compare the results with the PCA based segmentation method in [2]. Again, as mentioned before, our 2D-PCA based framework outperforms the conventional PCA as shown in Fig. 9a. Additionally, Fig. 9b studies the effect of choosing the number of the projected training shapes N (see Sect. 2) on the segmentation accuracy. From

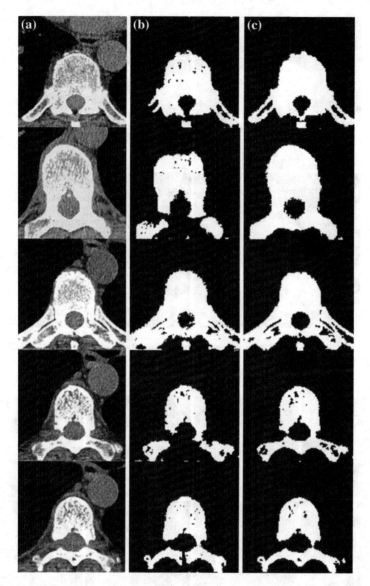

Fig. 6 Comparison between the intensity based segmentation (initial labeling) using: **a** Region of interest (after matched filter), **b** Scalar level sets model [8], and **c** Tensor level sets model [14]

this figure, we can conclude that the performance of 2D-PCA is better than the conventional PCA under the same number of training shapes. In another word, to get the same accuracy of PCA framework, the 2D-PCA needs fewer training shapes.

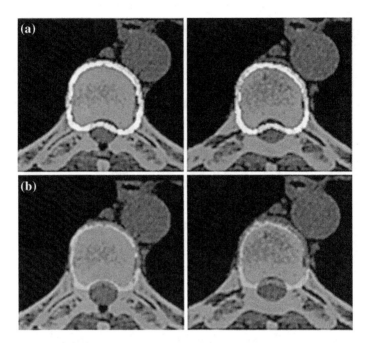

Fig. 7 Segmentation results of three different methods: (**a**) Method described in [2], and (**b**) Our 2D-PCA based segmentation

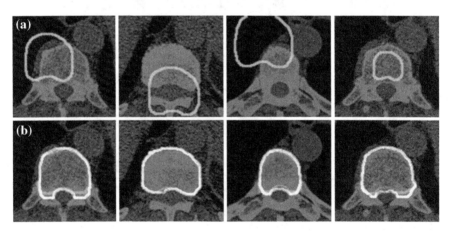

Fig. 8 Segmentation results with various shape initialization. (**a**) the initial shape prior, and (**b**) is the final results. The *red* and *yellow colors* show the contour of the gold standards and segmented regions

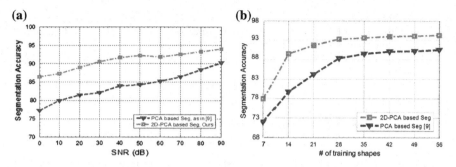

Fig. 9 **a** The average segmentation accuracy of different segmentation methods on 1400 CT images under various signal-to-noise ratios. **b** The effect of choosing the number of the projected training shapes N on the segmentation accuracy

4 Conclusions and Future Work

In this paper, we propose a new shape based segmentation of VBs in clinical CT images. Our method adopts the tensor level sets model for initial labeling and 2D-PCA for the shape prior construction. Validity was analyzed using ground truths of clinical datasets as well as the Europe-an Spine Phantom (ESP). The experimental results show that the noise immunity and the segmen-tation accuracy of our approach are much higher than conventional approaches. On the other hand, the tensor level sets representation is still computationally inefficient compared to the scalar level set. Future directions are geared towards speeding up our framework by adopting modern graphics processing units (GPUs) in the segmentation step.

References

1. Abdelmunim, H., Farag, A.A.: Curve/surface representation and evolution using vector level sets with application to the shape-based pattern analysis and machine intelligence. IEEE Trans. 29(6) (2007)
2. Aslan, M.S., Abdelmunim, H., Farag, A.A., Arnold, B., Mustafa, E., Xiang, P.: A new shape based segmentation framework using statistical and variational methods. In: Proceedings of IEEE International Conference on Image Processing (ICIP) (2011)
3. Aslan, M.S., Ali, A., Chen, D., Arnold, B., Farag, A.A., Xiang, P.: 3D vertebrae segmentation using graph cuts with shape prior constraints. In: Proceedings of IEEE International Conference on Image Processing (ICIP) (2010)
4. Aslan, M.S., Ali, A., Farag, A.A., Abdelmunim, H., Arnold, B., Xiang, P.: A new segmenta-tion and registration approach for vertebral body analysis. Proceedings of IEEE International Symposium on Biomedical Imaging (ISBI) (2011)
5. Aslan, M.S., Ali, A., Farag, A.A., Arnold, B., Chen, D., Xiang P.: 3D vertebrae segmentation in CT images with random noises. In: Proceedings of the International Conference on Pattern Recognition (ICPR'10) (2010)
6. Aslan, M.S., Ali, A., Rara, H., Arnold, B., Farag, A.A., Fahmi, R., Xiang, P.: A novel 3D segmentation of vertebral bones from volumetric CT images using graph cuts. ISVC'09 (2009)

7. Aslan, M.S., Mostafa, E., Abdelmunim, H., Shalaby, A., Farag, A.A., Arnold, B.: A novel probabilistic simultaneous segmentation and registration using level set. Proceedings of the International Conference on Image Processing (ICIP) (2011)

8. Chen, T.F., Vese, L.A.: Active contours without edge. IEEE Trans. Image Process. **10**(2), 266–277 (2001)

9. Kalender, W.A., Felsenberg, D., Genant, H., Fischer, M., Dequeker, J., Reeve, J.: The European spine phantom–a tool for standardization and quality control in spinal bone measurements by DXA and QCT. J. Radiol. **20**, 83–92 (1995)

10. Kaminsky, J., Klinge, P., Bokemeyer, M., Luedemann, W., Samii, M.: Specially adapted interactive tools for an improved 3D-segmentation of the spine. Comput. Med. Imaging Graph. **28**(3), 118–127 (2004)

11. Kang, Y., Engelke, K., Kalender, W.A.: New accurate and precise 3D segmentation method for skeletal structures in volumetric CT data. IEEE Trans. Med. Imaging (TMI) **22**(5), 586–598 (2003)

12. Mastmeyer, A., Engelke, K., Fuchs, C., Kalender, W.A.: A hierarchical 3D segmentation method and the definition of vertebral body coordinate systems for QCT of the lumbar spine. Med. Image Anal. **10**(4), 560–577 (2006)

13. Shalaby, A., Mahmoud, A., Mostafa, E., Abdoulmalek, A., Farag, A.A.: Segmentation framework of vertebral body using 2D-PCA. In: Proceedings of 15th Saudi Technical Exchange Meeting, (STEM'12), Dhahran, Saudi Arabia, pp. 81–85. 17–19 Dec 2012

14. Wang, B., Gao, X., Tao, D., Li, X.: A unified tensor level set for image segmentation. IEEE Trans. Syst. Man Cybern. **40**(3), 857–867 (2010)

15. Yang, J., Zhang, D., Frangi, A.F., Yang, J.: Two-dimensional PCA: a new approach to appearance based face representation and recognition. IEEE Trans. Pattern Anal. Mach. Intell. **26**(1), 131–137 (2004)

Part II
Computer Aided Detection and Diagnosis

Computer Aided Detection of Spinal Degenerative Osteophytes on Sodium Fluoride PET/CT

Jianhua Yao, Hector Munoz, Joseph E. Burns, Le Lu
and Ronald M. Summers

Abstract Osteophytes, a common degenerative change in the spine, are found in 90 % of the population over 60 years of age. We have developed an automated system to detect and assess spinal osteophytes on ^{18}F-sodium fluoride (^{18}F-NaF) PET/CT studies. We first segment the cortical shell of the vertebral body and unwrap it to a 2D map. Multiple characteristic features derived from PET/CT images are then projected onto the map. Finally, we adopt a three-tier learning based scheme to compute a confidence map and detect osteophyte sites and clusters. The system was tested on 20 studies (10 training and 10 testing) and achieved 84 % sensitivity at 3.8 false positives per case for the training set, and 82 % sensitivity at a 4.7 false positive rate for the testing set.

1 Introduction

Degenerative disc disease (DDD) develops with degeneration of the nucleus pulposus of the intervertebral discs (IVD) of the spine. As the nucleus pulposus desiccates, its volume, height, and elasticity are reduced and the IVD loses its ability to stably support loads. Spinal osteophytes are abnormal bony outgrowths that form along the disc margins in response to degenerative changes in the IVD and the associated altered biomechanics between the vertebral bodies. This osteophyte development occurs at the intervertebral interspaces and can inhibit normal spinal motion as well

J. Yao (✉) · H. Munoz · L. Lu · R. M. Summers
Radiology and Imaging Sciences Department, Clinical Center National Institutes of Health,
Bethesda, MD20892, USA
e-mail: jyao@cc.nih.gov

J. E. Burns
Department of Radiological Sciences, University of California, Irvine School of Medicine,
Orange, CA, USA
e-mail: jburns@uci.edu

J. Yao et al. (eds.), *Computational Methods and Clinical Applications*
for Spine Imaging, Lecture Notes in Computational Vision and Biomechanics 17,
DOI: 10.1007/978-3-319-07269-2_5, © Springer International Publishing Switzerland 2014

as progress to complete osseous bridging that fuses vertebrae. Osteophytes become more prevalent in the spine with increasing age, and are found in 90 % of population over 60 years old [1].

Investigations into computer-aided evaluation of spinal pathology and condition have been limited. The main areas of focus to date have involved spine lesions, scoliosis, fractures, and morphological change. There have been a few prior works targeting degenerative change and spinal osseous excrescences. Tan et al. [2] sought to quantitatively measure the status of ankylosing spondylitis via the segmentation of individual vertebra with successive level sets, followed by the segmentation of bony outgrowths (syndesmophytes) and quantification of their volume and height. Another method [3] dealt directly with detection of osteophytosis in the spine using radiographs of the cervical spine to detect and classify types of anterior osteophytes. Herrmann et al. [4] tracked the time variation of vertebral morphology between radiographs due to degenerative changes. While these methods focus on osseous excrescences which can be secondary indicators of DDD, other methods have focused directly on the IVD themselves. One method detected degenerating IVDs on MRI using 2D methods that analyzed disc intensity, location, and spacing [5]. A more recent approach segmented both the vertebral bodies and IVDs to detect degenerating IVDs in asymptomatic patients [6].

Degenerative osteophytes present in a variety of sizes, shapes, and densities, some examples of which are shown in Fig. 1, and can sometimes mimic the appearance of other pathologic processes. Osteophytes can be differentiated,in part, from dense regions of the spine of alternative etiology, by their spatial localization to the cortical shell of vertebra. They often form oblique longitudinal patterns across many verte-bral bodies, following the distribution of biomechanical load stressors as modified by physiologic homeostatic processes. CT imaging is useful to detect these osteo-phytes, diagnosed as marginal regions of dysmorphic cortical shell thickening of the vertebral bodies, typically (but not universally) with a higher X-ray attenuation than the adjacent cortex. Additionally, on physiologic imaging modalities, osteophytes may manifest with increased activity due to processes such as active mineraliza-tion, induced by mechanical stressors and associated progressive exostosis. Unfor-tunately, actively mineralizing bone, which has preferential uptake in ^{18}F-sodium fluoride (^{18}F-NaF) PET can be found in both osteophytes and metastases. Thus, osteophytes and spine metastases can manifest with similar and overlapping appear-ances on CT and ^{18}F-NaF PET images. Our goal is to explore the set of multimodal imaging features of osteophytes on PET and CT, characterizing both physiological and morphological elements, to search for and incorporate synergistic combinations of these features into a CAD system that can automatically detect spinal osteophytes on ^{18}F-NaF PET/CT.

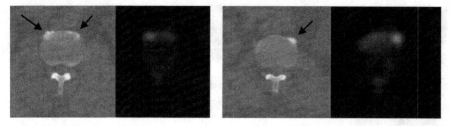

Fig. 1 Examples of osteophytes (*arrows*) on axial CT (*left*) and PET (*right*) images at two different vertebral levels

2 Methods and Material

Data: With IRB approval, we collected 20 ^{18}F-NaF PET/CT scans from 20 patients. The study population consisted of 15 males and 5 females, with a mean age of 64 ± 10. All patients were scanned on a Philips GEMINI TF scanner. Doses ranging from 112×10^6 to 203×10^6 Bq/ml of ^{18}F-NaF were administered intravenously to the patients, followed by physiologic uptake periods ranging from 114 to 126 min prior to image acquisition. The axial PET images were 144×144 or 169×169 pixels, at an axial spatial resolution of 4 mm $\times$ 4 mm per pixel and 4 mm slice spacing. Corresponding low dose technique of CT scanning was also performed. The scanning parameters for CT were: 5 mm slice thickness, 120 kVp, no intravenous contrast administration, and convolution kernel B. An experienced radiologist manually annotated the location of osteophyte sites on each CT slice (shown in Fig. 4).

2.1 Method Overview

For a given PET/CT data set, the PET data is first resampled to have the same resolution as the CT data. The spine is segmented on the CT images. The cortical shell of vertebral body is then extracted and unwrapped to a 2D map. Morphological and physiological features derived from both CT and PET are projected onto the map. A three-tier classification scheme is then applied to detect spinal degenerative osteophytes. The annotated location markers for the osteophytes are used as the reference standard to train the classifiers at each stage.

2.2 Spinal Segmentation and Cortical Shell Unwrapping

Spine segmentation is accomplished through thresholding, fuzzy connectivity and anatomical vertebral models. The spinal canal is first extracted using a directed graph search. Then a vertebral template is fit along the spinal canal. Finally, the spinal col-

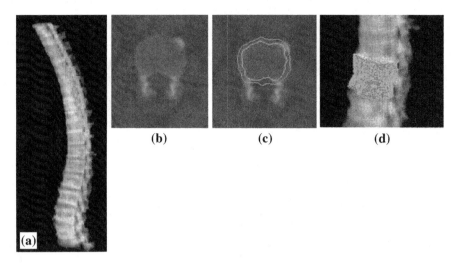

Fig. 2 Spine and cortical shell segmentation. **a** Spine segmentation result. *Red line*: centerline of spinal canal; **b** one cross section of the vertebra; **c** cortical shell segmentation at one cross section, *cyan*: periosteal surface, *red*: endosteal surface. **d** 3D surface of the cortical shell segmentation

umn is partitioned into vertebrae by detecting the IVD on curved planar reformations in sagittal and coronal directions. Details of the automated spinal column extraction and partitioning can be found in [7]. Figure 2a shows the segmented spine.

Since degenerative osteophytes occur at the cortical shell of the vertebral body, we apply a deformable dual-surface model to extract the periosteal and endosteal surfaces of the cortical shell at each vertebral level. The initial model consists of two concentric cylinders with their axes aligned with vertebral body axis and radii twice the average radius of vertebral bodies. The surface is represented as $r = S(z, \varphi)$ in the cylindrical coordinate system, where z is the distance along the axis, φ is the azimuth angle, and r is the radial distance. The vertices on the surface are then denoted as $(r\cos\varphi, r\sin\varphi, z)$. The periosteal and endosteal surfaces are represented as $r = S_p(z, \varphi)$ and $r = S_e(z, \varphi)$ respectively. The dual-surface is driven by the synergy of internal force, image force and constraint between the two surfaces, written as,

$$E(S) = w_i D(S) + w_p P(S) + w_c C(S_p, S_e) \tag{1}$$

where the internal forces $D(S)$ are spline forces derived from partial differential geometry that keep the surface smooth and continuous. The potential forces $P(S)$ are derived from the directional gradient along the radial direction of the cylindrical coordinate system. The dual-surface constraint ensures thickness transitions smoothly over the cortical shell, written as,

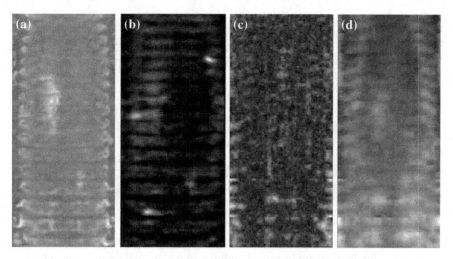

Fig. 3 Stacked feature maps of cortical shell for the entire spine. Each strip represents one vertebra. **a** Mean CT density map; **b** SUV max map; **c** thickness map; and **d** radius map

$$C(S_p, S_e) = \int \left(\left| \frac{\partial (S_p(z, \varphi) - S_e(z, \varphi))}{\partial z} + \frac{\partial (S_p(z, \varphi) - S_e(z, \varphi))}{\partial \varphi} \right| \right) dz d\varphi \quad (2)$$

The weights for different forces (w_i, w_p and w_c) in Eq. 1 are kept constant throughout the evolution. Figure 2b–d shows the result of cortical shell segmentation.

The unwrapping of the cortical shell is based on the cylindrical coordinate system. We map the 3D cortical shell between the two surfaces onto the 2D space of (z, φ), written as,

$$R(S_p(z, \varphi), S_e(z, \varphi)) \rightarrow U(z, \varphi) \quad (3)$$

where $R(\ )$ is the feature function to be projected. The mapping is one-to-one, i.e., every point on the cortical shell corresponds to one point on the map. The horizontal axis is φ and the vertical axis is z. Axis φ starts from the center of the spinal canal and spans 360°, and axis z goes from the inferior to the superior endplates. We then stack the map of each vertebra body to form the whole map for the entire spine column. The individual vertebra maps are naturally aligned through the spinal canal. Examples of the unwrapped spine maps are in Fig. 3. More information about the cortical shell unwrapping can be found in [8].

2.3 Characteristic Feature Map Computation

Through the unwrapping operation, we effectively convert the complex 3D detection problem into a 2D problem. Multiple features from CT and PET are projected to the 2D map to characterize the morphological, textural and physiological properties of the cortical shell. The following feature maps are generated,

1. Thickness: $U_1(z, \varphi) = S_p(z, \varphi) - S_e(z, \varphi)$
2. Radius: $U_2(z, \varphi) = S_p(z, \varphi)$
3. Mean density: $U_3(z, \varphi) = \frac{1}{U_1(z,\varphi)} \int_{S_e(z,\varphi)}^{S_p(z,\varphi)} I(z, \varphi, r) dr$
4. Max density: $U_4(z, \varphi) = \max_{r=S_e(z,\varphi)}^{S_p(z,\varphi)} (I(z, \varphi, r))$
5. Interior density: $U_5(z, \varphi) = \frac{1}{S_e(z,\varphi)} \int_0^{S_e(z,\varphi)} I(z, \varphi, r) dr$
6. Exterior density: $U_6(z, \varphi) = \frac{1}{S_e(z,\varphi)} \int_{S_p(z,\varphi)}^{S_p(z,\varphi)+S_e(z,\varphi)} I(z, \varphi, r) dr$
7. Mean SUV: $U_7(z, \varphi) = \frac{1}{U_1(z,\varphi)} \int_{S_e(z,\varphi)}^{S_p(z,\varphi)} SUV(z, \varphi, r) dr$
8. Max SUV: $U_8(z, \varphi) = \max_{r=S_e(z,\varphi)}^{S_p(z,\varphi)} (SUV(z, \varphi, r))$
9. Interior SUV: $U_9(z, \varphi) = \frac{1}{S_e(z,\varphi)} \int_0^{S_e(z,\varphi)} SUV(z, \varphi, r) dr$
10. Exterior SUV: $U_{10}(z, \varphi) = \frac{1}{S_e(z,\varphi)} \int_{S_p(z,\varphi)}^{S_p(z,\varphi)+S_e(z,\varphi)} SUV(z, \varphi, r) dr$

Here $I()$ is the CT value, and $SUV()$ is the standardized uptake value from PET, which is normalized for dose and body mass. Examples of feature maps are shown in Fig. 3.

2.4 Three-Tier Classification Scheme

The detection of potential osteophytes is conducted on the multi-channel feature map of the cortical shell by a robust three-tier supervised learning system. First, a region covariance descriptor is applied to compute the confidence map of the occurrence. In the second stage, a multi-channel feature vector is computed for each point on the cortical shell and employed to detect the osteophyte sites at each cross section. In the third stage, the osteophyte sites are clustered and characteristic features are computed for the final classification.

Confidence map generation using covariance descriptor: Region covariance descriptor [9] is adopted to capture the statistical appearance correlations among osteophyte regions, and to compute the confidence of osteophyte occurrence. The operation is conducted on the mean density map (U_3). The feature vector for each point (z, φ) on the map is, $F(z, \varphi) = \{z, \varphi, U_3(z, \varphi), |\partial_z U_3|, |\partial_\varphi U_3|, |\partial_z^2 U_3|, |\partial_\varphi^2 U_3|, |\partial_z U_3^s|, |\partial_\varphi U_3^s|, |\partial_z^2 U_3^s|, |\partial_\varphi^2 U_3^s|\}$ here U_3^s is the Gaussian smoothed image of U_3. The resulting feature covariance matrix C is 11×11 and has 66 independent parameters due to symmetry. From the manual markers (Fig. 4a), we can obtain two sets of positive $\{C^+\}$ and negative $\{C^-\}$ samples for training. Although the distance between any pair (C_1, C_2) is defined on a Riemannian manifold as $d(C1, C2) = \sqrt{\sum_{i=1}^{11} ln^2 \lambda_i(C_1, C_2)}$, we can formulate a new Mercer kernel $K(C_1, C_2) = \exp(-d(C_1, C_2)/\sigma)$ to train a support vector machine (SVM) because $d(C_1, C_2)$ is a metric. λ_i is the generalized eigenvalue of $eig(C_1, C_2)$ and σ is calibrated as the mean of $d(C_1, C_2)$ from $\{C^+\}$ and $\{C^-\}$. In runtime, we evaluate each $N \times N$ scanning window ($N = 25$) centered every 3 pixels in z and φ direction, using the trained classifier. If classified as positive, every pixel inside the window

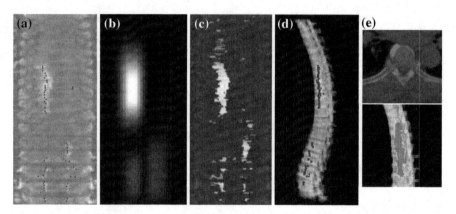

Fig. 4 Three-tier classification. **a** Reference standard projected onto the stacked feature map (*red dots*); **b** confidence map; **c** detected ostephyte sites, highlighted horizontal segments; and **d** final detections projected back to 3D spine, *red*: reference standard,, *blue*: detections; **e** osteophyte cluster detection on 2D and 3D display

gets one count so that the accumulated count map represents the overall confidence level of prior detection. Fig. 4b shows an example of the confidence map.

Osteophyte site detection: An osteophyte site is defined as a span of osteophytes on a cross-section of a vertebra, which appears as a horizontal segment on the feature map. The detection process is as follows: (1) the initial seeds (z_s, φ_s) are identified at the local maximum in a 7×1 window on the mean density map (U_3); (2) the seeds are extended to horizontal segments; and (3) feature vectors are computed for each segment and used for classification.

To extend a seed point (z_s, φ_s) to a segment (L, R), where $L = (z_s, \varphi_L)$ and $R = (z_s, \varphi_R)$ are border points on each side, we first compute the background density $B(z_s)$ at each cross section z_s. The mean density of the lower 50 % is used as the background. The border points are then located at the half maximum between the seed point density and background density. That is, φ_L is the largest φ where $\varphi < \varphi_S$ and $U_3(z_s, \varphi) < (U_3(z_s, \varphi_s) + B(z_s))/2$. Similarly, φ_R can be located.

The segments (L, R) are then treated as potential osteophyte sites. For a site, a feature vector of $(\overline{U_1}, \overline{U_2}, \ldots \overline{U_{10}}, p)$ is computed, where $\overline{U_k}$ is the mean feature value of map k for all points in the segment, and p is the mean confidence value from the confidence map.

A SVM classifier is generated using the reference markers by radiologists. The markers are first mapped to the cortical shell map (Fig. 4a). Then, the mapped markers are extended to segments, and feature vectors are assigned. Other local maxima not including the reference markers are treated as false samples for the classifier training. The osteophyte sites passing the classifier are then sent to the next phase of further classification.

Osteophyte clustering: One characteristic feature of degenerative change is that the osteophytes often form oblique longitudinal patterns across many vertebral bodies.

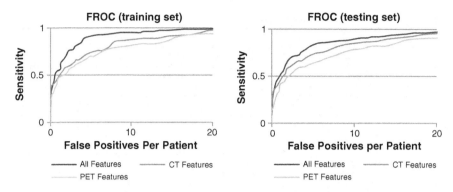

Fig. 5 FROC analysis

We capture this feature by clustering of osteophytesites based on their spatial connectivity, with each cluster treated as one osteophyte detection. We then compute the morphological, textural, physiological, and location features for each detection. The morphological features include height, width, and thickness. The textural features include mean and standard deviation of density, and the contrast between the detection and its neighborhood (both circumferential and radial neighbors). Location features include circumferential location, distance to pedicle, and distance to IVD. One important feature is to count the detections within a limited range of circumferential locations (φ) about an osteophyte site, with more occurrences within that range boosting the probability of the initial osteophyte site being a true osteophyte. We then form another SVM classifier using the cluster features to get the final detection (Fig. 4d, e).

3 Experimental Results

We divided our data into independent training and testing sets, with 10 studies in each set. The numbers of osteophytes larger than 5mm were 100 and 97 in the training and testing sets, respectively. The performance of our system was evaluated using FROC analysis. If a reference marker was within the detections, it was treated as a detected osteophyte; otherwise it was a false negative. If a detection covered at least one reference marker, it was a true positive, otherwise a false positive. We conducted the classification using all features, CT features only, and PET features only (Fig. 5). In the training set, the sensitivities (FP rates) were 84 % (3.8), 80 % (7.3), and 80 % (9.6) for all features, CT features, and PET features respectively. In the testing set, the sensitivities (FP rates) were 82 % (4.7), 81 % (8.0), and 79 % (10.9) respectively. The performance differences (false positive rate) between using all features and CT or PET features alone were statistically significant ($p < 0.001$, Fisher Exact test).

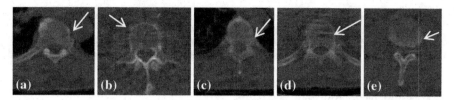

Fig. 6 Examples of false negatives (**a, b**) and false positives (**c, d, e**)

Figure 6 shows examples of false negatives and false positives. The etiology of missed osteophytes includes influences from other lesions on the same vertebra (a) and image artifact (b). The etiology of common false positives includes costovertebral junction (c), image artifact (d) and partial volume averaging of IVDs (e).

4 Discussion

Assessment of spine osteophytes has significant potential for clinical application. It is a valuable indicator of spine degeneration and can be used to monitor the progress of treatment or disease. Since our technique is automatic and efficient, it can run in background to assess the osteophyte burden for every PET/CT or CT data set. This is the first CAD system for spinal osteophytes with sufficient performance.

The low-dose low-resolution technique of CT scanning in PET/CT creates numerous challenges to the segmentation of vertebrae and their cortical shell unwrapping. We address this problem with a dual-surface deformable model constrained by anatomical shape. The synergistic multi-modality feature integration of PET and CT features captures the attributes of degenerative change that one modality alone cannot. For instance, while both degenerative disease and metastases can demonstrate increased ^{18}F-NaF uptake on PET imaging, some manifestations of degenerative osteophytosis are not as hyperdense as sclerotic metastatic disease on the CT. Combining PET and CT, other morphological features can also differentiate these entities. Future plans include further development of this system to assist in the differentiation of degenerative osteophytes and metastatic bone lesions.

Acknowledgments This work was supported by the Intramural Research Program at National Institutes of Health, Clinical Center.

References

1. Nathan, H.: Osteophytes of the vertebral column an anatomical study of their development according to age, race, and sex with considerations as to their etiology and significance. J. Bone Joint Surg. **44**, 243–268 (1962)
2. Tan, S., Yao, J., Ward, M.: Computer aided evaluation of ankylosing spondylitis using high-resolution CT. IEEE Trans. Med. Imaging **27**(9), 1252–1267 (2008)

3. Stanley, R.J., et al.: Size-invariant descriptors for detecting regions of abnormal growth in cervical vertebrae. Comput. Med. Imaging Graph. **32**(1), 44–52 (2008)
4. Herrmann, A.M., Geisler, F.H.: A new computer-aided technique for analysis of lateral cervical radiographs in postoperative patients with degenerative disease. Spine **29**(16), 1795–1803 (2004)
5. Alomari, R.S., et al.: Computer-aided diagnosis of lumbar disc pathology from clinical lower spine MRI. Int. J. CARS **5**, 287–293 (2010)
6. Neubert, A., Fripp, J.: Automated detection, 3D segmentation and analysis of high resolution spine MR images using statistical shape models. Phys. Med. **57**(24), 8357–8375 (2012)
7. Yao, J., O'Connor, S., Summers, R.M.: Extraction, automated spinal column, partitioning. In: IEEE ISBI. Arlington, Virginia, USA (2006)
8. Yao, J., et al.: Detection of vertebral body fractures based on cortical shell unwrapping. MICCAI **3**, 509–516 (2012)
9. Tuzel, O., Porikli, F., Meer, P.: Pedestrian detection via classification on Riemannian manifolds. IEEE Trans. Pattern Anal. Mach. Intell. **30**(10), 1713–1727 (2008)

Novel Morphological and Appearance Features for Predicting Physical Disability from MR Images in Multiple Sclerosis Patients

Jeremy Kawahara, Chris McIntosh, Roger Tam and Ghassan Hamarneh

Abstract Physical disability in patients with multiple sclerosis is determined by functional ability and quantified with numerical scores. In vivo studies using magnetic resonance imaging (MRI) have found that these scores correlate with spinal cord atrophy (loss of tissue), where atrophy is commonly measured by spinal cord volume or cross-sectional area. However, this correlation is generally weak to moderate, and improved measures would strengthen the utility of imaging biomarkers. We propose novel spinal cord morphological and MRI-based appearance features. Select features are used to train regression models to predict patients' physical disability scores. We validate our models using 30 MRI scans of different patients with varying levels of disability. Our results suggest that regression models trained with multiple spinal cord features predict clinical disability better than a model based on the volume of the spinal cord alone.

1 Introduction

Multiple sclerosis (MS) studies have found that a patient's physical disability correlates with spinal cord atrophy [1, 7, 8, 12, 16]. Measuring spinal cord atrophy is potentially useful for monitoring the progression of diseases or the effectiveness

J. Kawahara (✉) · C. McIntosh · G. Hamarneh
Medical Image Analysis Lab., Simon Fraser University, Burnaby, Canada
e-mail: jkawahar@sfu.ca

C. McIntosh
Princess Margaret Cancer Centre, University Health Network, Toronto, Canada
e-mail: Chris.McIntosh@rmp.uhn.on.ca

R. Tam
MS/MRI Research Group, University of British Columbia, Vancouver, Canada
e-mail: roger.tam@ubc.ca

G. Hamarneh
e-mail: hamarneh@sfu.ca

J. Yao et al. (eds.), *Computational Methods and Clinical Applications
for Spine Imaging*, Lecture Notes in Computational Vision and Biomechanics 17,
DOI: 10.1007/978-3-319-07269-2_6, © Springer International Publishing Switzerland 2014

of therapies [12]. Spinal cord atrophy is defined as a loss of tissue and commonly measured by cross-sectional area (CSA) or spinal cord volume [7, 8, 12]. To quantify the CSA, user-guided computer software is often used to assist in delineating the spinal cord from a 3D MRI (e.g. using one of several recently developed approaches [4, 5, 10, 11, 15]). The segmented cord's volume or averaged CSA is computed and correlated with the patient's clinical disability score.

To quantify the clinical disability of a patient with MS, clinicians commonly rely on the Expanded Disability Status Scale (EDSS) [6] which assigns the patient a number between zero (a normal neurological exam) and ten (death from MS). Although commonly used, the EDSS score suffers from reproducibility issues, focuses largely on a patient's ambulatory impairment, and is restricted to an ordinal scale. This motivated the development of the Multiple Sclerosis Functional Composite (MSFC) score [3], which we discuss in Sect. 2.5.

While the CSA of the spinal cord has been shown to correlate with clinical score, this correlation is generally moderate with some studies failing to show the expected reduction in CSA [9]. This may be because a reduction in cord size is only one global aspect of atrophy, and few other features that capture more subtle aspects have been explored. Schnabel et al. [13] explored local and global shape measurements across scales and concluded that the spinal cord shape should be measured across a range of scales. In conventional and diffusion tensor (DT) MRIs, Benedetti et al. [1] identified the brain T2 lesion volume, CSA and the mean fractional anisotropy of the cervical cord as features that independently influenced the EDSS score using a multivariate regression model. Composite scores, obtained by combining these three features, improved the correlation with clinical scores when compared to the correlations of a single feature. However, DT-MRI is much less commonly acquired than structural MRI. Valsasina et al. [16] explored the regional atrophy of the cervical cord by applying voxel-wise statistics on registered spinal cord segmentations. They used the determined regional atrophy in a multiple regression model, adjusted for age, sex, and cord volume, and showed correlations with clinical scores and patterns of atrophy.

Although a number of composite MRI biomarkers for MS have been proposed, computing morphological features to capture atrophy and combining these features in *linear* and *non-linear regression models* has not been well studied. As well, few works have testing whether combining *multiple spinal cord features* into a single model will provide a better indicator of disability than just using a single feature. Introducing new atrophic features and methods to combine them may assist clinicians in diagnosis, provide insights into disease progression, and serve as a useful composite biomarker.

We propose novel features extracted from MRI and the corresponding spinal cord segmentation that are potentially more specific to the clinical status than pure area or volume. Using these extracted features, we employ different regression models ranging in complexity and intuitiveness, starting with simple linear regression models, then multiple linear regression models and finally, non-linear non-parametric regression forests. To determine which of our proposed candidate features are useful biomarkers, we explore our data for features that are consistently associated with clinical state. Our results suggest that our proposed features and the more complex regression models are capable of outperforming the predictive abilities of a linear regression model using only spinal cord volume as the explanatory variable.

2 Methods

In this section we describe our data and the regression problem, examine the new candidate spinal cord features, outline the different types of regression models used, describe our cross-validation set-up, and finally discuss how the clinical scores are computed.

2.1 The Data and the Problem

We are given a set of n MRI scans $I = \{I_1, \ldots, I_n\}$ where each 3D MRI scan I_i has a corresponding real number clinical score $y_i \in Y$, and a corresponding spinal cord segmentation $S_i \in S$. The dimensions of I_i and S_i are the same. Each voxel in S_i has a value between 0 and 1, where 0 represents the background and 1 represents the spinal cord. Voxels in S_i that are on the boundary of the spinal cord are assigned a fuzzy value between 0 and 1 that represents an estimated percentage of the voxel that contains spinal cord (i.e., partial volume) [15].

Our objective is to create a model M, using the images I and segmentations S, capable of predicting the patients' clinical scores Y from novel MR images. We extract a set of features X from I and S that are transformed by model M into values $\hat{Y}$, such that these predicted values $\hat{Y} = M(X)$ estimate the corresponding clinical scores Y.

One approach is to set M as a simple linear regression model with the spinal cord volume as the single explanatory variable X. This is similar to the existing literature where a Pearson's correlation coefficient is computed to measure the linear dependency between the spinal cord volume and clinical score. However, as mentioned in the introduction, this linear dependency using spinal cord volume does not always reveal a strong clinical relationship. We improve on this by deriving new morphological and MRI-based appearance features X and examining ways to combine them in more descriptive models M.

2.2 Candidate Features

We describe simple candidate morphological and appearance features X that are potentially sensitive to spinal cord changes. This is not meant to be a comprehensive set of features, but is sufficient to explore the potential of going beyond measuring cord size to predict disability. We first define the commonly used spinal cord volume,

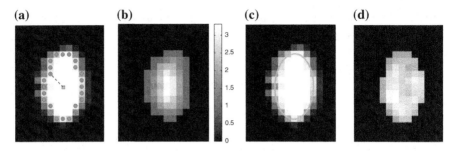

Fig. 1 Illustrations of the proposed features. **a** The distances (*dashed line*) from the center-of-mass (*center box*) to the boundary voxels (*circles*) make up per_k. **b** The distances to the nearest boundary point from the voxels inside the cord give $dist_k$ (brighter implies farther). **c** An ellipse is fit to the cord. **d** The normalized intensities of the cord are considered in int_k

which is computed by summing all voxels, including the partial volumes $S_i(j) \in [0, 1]$, in the segmentation, $vol = \sum_{j=1}^{J} S_i(j)$, where J is the total number of voxels in S_i. While spinal cord volume captures a global measure of spinal cord atrophy, we are also interested in features that vary at least partly independently from area or volume, and that are sensitive to spinal cord changes at a local scale.

Our first proposed feature is designed to be more sensitive to local changes in the spinal cord's boundary. On each 2D axial slice of the segmentation S_i, we find voxels on the boundary between the spinal cord and background by considering voxels in S_i with a partial volume greater than 0.5 to be spinal cord. This results in a 2D binary image that we use to extract the cord's boundary voxels. For the kth 2D axial slice of the spinal cord, we take the Euclidean distance between the center-of-mass c_k of the cord's kth cross section, and the spinal cord boundary/perimeter voxels b computed as, $per_k = (d(c_k, b_k^1), \ldots, d(c_k, b_k^{m(k)}))$, where b_k^i represents the ith boundary voxel on the kth slice, and $d(c, b)$ computes the Euclidean distance between the two coordinates (Fig. 1a). The number of boundary voxels $m(k)$ can change for each 2D slice. We find the *minimum* distance from the center-of-mass to the boundary voxels in each 2D slice averaged over K 2D slices,

$$per_{\min} = \frac{1}{K} \sum_{k=1}^{K} \min(per_k). \tag{1}$$

In a similar way, to compute additional features we replace the "min" function from (1) with the mean (per_{mean}), standard deviation (per_{std}), and the max ($per_{\max}$) functions.

We define a related measure that focuses on local changes in 3D by calculating a 3D distance transform from the surface of the segmented spinal cord masked by (or restricted to) the interior region of the cord. To compute the distance transform, we calculate the Euclidean distance between voxels inside the spinal cord and the nearest boundary voxel in 3D. To further differentiate this feature from the *per* features, we consider voxels that contain any partial volume to be spinal cord, which changes the boundary voxels. The distance transform for slice k with q voxels inside the cord is represented as $dist_k = (t_k^1, \ldots, t_k^{q(k)})$ where t_k^i is the distance from the ith voxel inside the cord on the kth slice to the nearest 3D boundary coordinate (Fig. 1b). The number of voxels inside the cord, $q(k)$, can change for each 2D slice. In a similar fashion to (1), we replace per_k with $dist_k$ and the "min" function with the mean ($dist_{mean}$), max ($dist_{max}$), standard deviation ($dist_{std}$) and the max divided by the mean distance ($dist_{mean}^{max}$) function averaged over the K 2D slices. For clarity we formally define,

$$dist_{mean}^{max} = \frac{1}{K} \sum_{k=1}^{K} \frac{\max(dist_k)}{\text{mean}(dist_k)}, \tag{2}$$

which averages the ratio of the furthest boundary distance by the mean distance.

To compute features that are more robust to local noise, such as small segmentation errors, we fit an ellipse (Fig. 1c) to each 2D cross-sectional slice of the segmented spinal cord and compute the eccentricity (ecc), minor axis (ax_{min}), and major axis (ax_{maj}), averaged over the length the cord.

All the features proposed so far are dependent on the geometrical characteristics of the cord, but we also include features based on the intensities found within the MRI. As the intensity values can vary widely in different MRI scans, we normalize a scan's intensities by its overall 3D scan intensities to produce z-scores. We extract the z-scores of those voxels that are labelled as spinal cord (partial volume > 0.5) and take the mean (int_{mean}) and standard deviation (int_{std}) of the spinal cord intensity values averaged over the K 2D slices (Fig. 1d).

2.3 Regression Models

Linear regression employs a linear function to model the relationship between the explanatory variable (e.g. spinal cord volume) and a response variable (clinical score). The parameters of this model are the coefficients β of the explanatory variables and the error term ε. These coefficients can be estimated from the data by applying a *least-squares* fitting that minimizes the differences between the response variable and the fitted explanatory variable. A model with only a single explanatory variable x_1, is known as *simple linear regression*, and is one of the simplest models to analyze. Given a dataset with n observations, this produces a straight line, $y_i = \beta_1 x_{i1} + \varepsilon_i, i = 1, \ldots, n$. *Multiple linear regression* builds on this by adding r explanatory variables to the model, $y_i = \beta_1 x_{i1} + \cdots + \beta_r x_{ir} + \varepsilon_i$.

While these models assume a linearity of the underlying relations, we also explore a more flexible, non-linear, non-parametric model, known as a *regression forest*. A regression forest significantly differs from the previously described models as it is completely learned from the data and makes no assumptions about the underlying distributions [2].

2.4 Training and Testing the Models

The models in Sect. 2.3, are described in order of increasing complexity. With this added complexity, we increase the potential to accurately model the underlying function, but also increase the difficulty in intuitively understanding the model and increase the likelihood of over-fitting the model to the training data. To reduce the possibility of over-fitting, we divide our data into a training and testing set. Given the relatively small size of our dataset, we use leave-one-out cross-validation. This is repeated for all samples to give us an indication of the robustness and generalizability of our regression model and chosen features.

2.5 Clinical Scores

As discussed in the introduction, the EDSS and the MSFC scores, which we aim to predict from X, are commonly used to quantify clinical disability. We choose to focus on the MSFC score rather than the EDSS score because the MSFC captures disability to which the EDSS score is relatively insensitive, such as arm/hand function. In addition, the EDSS scores tend to exhibit a poor distribution due to the non-linearity of the scale, with many patients clustered between 4.5 and 6.5 (Fig. 2a).

The MSFC score tests for: upper extremity function, determined by a 9-hole peg test (9-HPT); walking speed, measured by a timed 25-foot walk (T25W); and cognitive function, evaluated by a paced auditory serial addition test (PASAT). These three tests are shown to vary relatively independently, be sensitive to changes over time, and capture aspects of MS that are not captured in the EDSS score [3]. These components averaged together compose the MSFC score,

$$Z_{MSFC} = (Z_{9\text{-HPT}} - Z_{T25W} + Z_{PASAT})/3 \tag{3}$$

where the scores are normalized to produce z-scores using a reference population that includes healthy controls [3].

While this composite score is used to give an overall indication of the progression of multiple sclerosis, we do not expect the cognitive component, Z_{PASAT}, to have a strong causal relation with spinal cord atrophy as the spinal cord is not directly related to cognitive function. We test this by computing the Pearson's correlation coefficient with the cognitive test Z_{PASAT} and spinal cord volume vol, and do not find a significant correlation ($r = -0.016$, p-value $= 0.93$). For this reason, we remove Z_{PASAT} and only include the physical disability tests to define a new clinical measurement of physical disability,

$$Z_{physical} = (Z_{9\text{-HPT}} - Z_{T25W})/2. \tag{4}$$

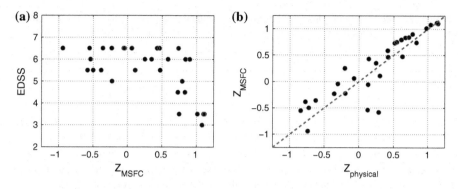

Fig. 2 The distributions of scores are shown. **a** The Z_{MSFC} scores have a wider distributions than EDSS scores. As expected, as EDSS decreases, there is a trend for Z_{MSFC} to increase. **b** We remove the cognitive component from Z_{MSFC} to form $Z_{physical}$, slightly changing the distributions (*deviations from dashed line*)

This combined physical score, $Z_{physical}$, is the clinical score we use as the response variable for this work. The distribution of values and the changes in correlation between Z_{MSFC} and $Z_{physical}$ are shown in Fig. 2b.

3 Results

We validate our proposed features and models using 30 3D T1-weighted MRIs acquired with a spoiled gradient echo sequence and an MR field strength of either 1.5 T or 3.0 T. These scans were gathered from multiple centers and parameters varied by site. Each scan is from a different patient (age ranged from 34 to 64) with secondary progressive MS. For each 3D MRI, we have its corresponding clinical score as described in Sect. 2.5 and a segmentation of the spinal cord. To ensure reasonably accurate segmentations, we use a seeded semi-automatic method similar to Tench et al. [15] where a user-guided region growing algorithm marks the spinal cord voxels with a 1 and the background voxels with a 0. Due to the limited resolution of the MRIs and the small size of the cord, voxels on the boundary of the spinal cord, composed both of spinal cord and background, make up approximately 25 % of the total voxels in the cross-sectional area [15]. To give an estimate of the spinal cord area contribution these boundary voxels make, the boundary voxels are assigned a fuzzy value between 0 and 1, computed as a function of the cord, boundary and cerebrospinal fluid intensities, based on Eq. (2) in [15]. The original MRI voxel resolutions were either $0.976 \times 0.976 \times 1$ mm or $0.976 \times 0.976 \times 1.3$ mm, but are normalized via trilinear interpolation to $1 \times 1 \times 1$ mm. When computing our features X, we only consider the first 20 2D slices starting from and including the C3 region and moving inferior, i.e. $K = 20$ in (1) and (2).

Table 1 The *model* column contains the different type of models explored where *linear* represents a linear model, *multiple* represents a multiple linear regression model, and *RF* represents a regression forest model

Model	Features	MAE	SAE	RMSE	r	p-value
Linear	vol	0.448	0.326	0.551	0.367	0.0460841
Linear	per_{min}	0.444	0.290	0.527	0.464	0.0097723
Multiple	$best_{7MR}$	0.379	0.253	0.453	0.667	0.0000565
Multiple	sel_{5MR}	0.414	0.233	0.473	0.617	0.0002851
RF	per_{min}	0.381	0.251	0.453	0.682	0.0000328
RF	sel_{2RF}	**0.293**	**0.201**	**0.353**	**0.803**	0.0000001

The *features* column contains the different features the model was trained on, where *vol* represents the volume of the spinal cord, per_{min} represents the minimal distance to the cord's center-of-mass from the cord's boundary, *best* represents the combination of features that gives the lowest RMSE error, and *sel* are the features consistently selected in our top 25 models. The error metrics we report are the Mean Absolute Error (MAE), the Root Mean Squared Error (RMSE), the Standard deviation of Absolute Error (SAE), the *Pearson's* correlation coefficient r and its corresponding p-value before correction for multiple comparisons

3.1 Error Metrics

To quantify how closely the predictions $\hat{Y}$ produced by our model are to the true clinical scores Y, we use the following metrics. We compute the *mean absolute error* (MAE) by taking the mean of the absolute difference between the predicted score and the true clinical score, $MAE = \frac{1}{n}\sum_i^n |\hat{y}_i - y_i|$, giving equal weight to all errors. To get an indication of the variability in the error, we compute the *standard deviation of absolute error* as, $SAE = std(|\hat{Y} - Y|)$. To give a higher weight to larger errors, we report the *root mean square error*, $RMSE = \sqrt{\frac{1}{n}\sum_i^n (\hat{y}_i - y_i)^2}$. MAE, SAE, and RMSE values closer to zero indicate a better model. To indicate the consistency of our predictions, we also compute the *Pearson's correlation coefficient* and its corresponding p-value between the predicted clinical scores $\hat{Y}$ and the true clinical scores Y.

3.2 Simple Linear Regression with Spinal Cord Volume

To establish a baseline test on which we aim to improve, we use a simple linear regression model with spinal cord volume as the explanatory variable similar to what is done by Losseff et al. [8]. We compute the volume of the segmented cord (*vol*) and use leave-out-one cross-validation to train our model and test on the omitted volume. As expected from the existing literature [1, 7, 8, 12, 16], we detect a moderate yet statistically significant correlation between volume and clinical score (*vol*: r = 0.473, $p = 0.00824$). The predictive ability for a linear regression model using volume as the explanatory variable is reported in Table 1 (row 1) and shown in Fig. 3a.

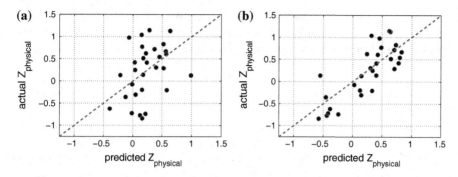

Fig. 3 Actual versus predicted clinical scores are shown. **a** Spinal cord volume *vol* is used as the explanatory variable in a simple linear regression model. **b** A regression forest trained on two selected features, ax_{maj} and per_{min}, demonstrates an improved correlation. Deviations from the *dashed line* are errors

3.3 Simple Linear Regression with Proposed Features

In our second test, we examine each proposed feature's ability to act as the explanatory variable in a linear model. For each proposed feature in Sect. 2.2, we compute the Pearson's correlation coefficient between the proposed feature and the clinical scores. We find that ax_{max}^{min}, per_{mean}, per_{min}, $dist_{max}^{mean}$ all provide a slight increase in correlation when compared to *vol*. Of these features, per_{min} shows the strongest improvement in Pearson's correlation (per_{min}: r $= 0.565$, $p = 0.00115$; vs. volume *vol*: r $= 0.473$, $p = 0.00824$) and the *p*-value of per_{min} survives the Bonferroni correction for multiple testing ($0.00115 < \frac{0.05}{13}$).

We test if per_{min} is a stronger explanatory variable than volume by performing the same cross-validation procedure. We report our results in Table 1 (row 2), which demonstrates that not only does per_{min} correlate better than volume, but it gives a more consistent score and is less susceptible to outliers. This is shown by the lower MAE, SAE, and RMSE scores, and higher Pearson's correlation when compared to a model using volume. This suggests that per_{min} may be a better indicator of physical disability than spinal cord volume.

3.4 Multiple Linear Regression with Proposed Features

To explore the use of multiple explanatory variables in a linear regression model, using the 13 candidate features described in Sect. 2.2, we form separate models where each feature can either be included or excluded from the model, for a total of $2^{13} = 8192$ possible combinations. To get a sense of which variables generalize well, we test each model using leave-one-out cross-validation. We correct for multiple testing by applying the positive False Discovery Rate (pFDR) [14] to reduce the likelihood that a positive result is a Type I error. As our goal is to determine if a multiple linear regression model can provide improvements over simple linear regression, we compute how many models result in a RMSE that are less than the RMSE reported using the linear model with the explanatory variable per_{min} (i.e. RMSE < 0.527). There are 292 such models and from this subset of models, we find the maximum p-value to be 0.00684 with a corresponding q-value of 0.00017. Out of all our tests, there are 749 tests with a p-value less than 0.00684, indicating a low number ($749 \times 0.00017 < 1$) of improved models that are potentially false positives. The features selected from the model with the lowest RMSE are: $best_{7MR}$ = $\{int_{mn}, ax_{min}, per_{mean}, per_{max}, per_{min}, dist_{max}, dist_{max}^{mean}\}$, and the prediction results are reported in Table 1 (row 3). We note that this model with multiple features shows a significant reduction in prediction error when compared to the models using a single explanatory variable.

However, as the issue of how best to correct for multiple testing is still an open one, we further examine our models for a more conservative selection of features. We examine what features were consistently selected in the top 25 models. As can been seen in Fig. 4, the same five features are selected in nearly every model suggesting these features jointly are useful. Based on this trend, we form a linear regression model using only the consistently selected features, sel_{5MR} = $\{int_{mean}, per_{mean}, per_{max}, dist_{max}, dist_{max}^{mean}\}$, and report the cross-validated results in Table 1 (row 4). While the predictive ability of this model is less than the $best_{7MR}$ predicting model, this model has two less explanatory variables than the $best_{7MR}$ model, which may be more generalizable in a novel dataset (even though we cross-validated our dataset). These improvements over the models with a single explanatory variable, suggests that it is useful to combine multiple spinal cord features within a single model.

3.5 Non-linear Regression Forest with Proposed Features

In our final tests, we use a non-linear regression forest (RF) implemented with MAT-LAB's TreeBagger class (R2012a; The MathWorks Inc., Natick, MA). The minimum number of observations per leaf is set to one. All other parameters are left to their default settings except for the number of trees which we describe below. To see if a non-linear model, trained on a single feature can outperform a linear model, we train a RF with 250 trees on each proposed feature from Sect. 2.2. Out of our 13 proposed features, we find that per_{min} on its own returns superior results when compared to the other models that use only a single feature, Table 1 (row 5). To consider multiple features in our RF, as was done in Sect. 3.4, we try all possible combinations of features (2^{13}) in a RF. However, to lower computational cost, we use 80 trees with 6-fold (instead of leave-one-out) cross validation when exploring all the feature combinations. We find those features used in the model that produces the lowest RMSE. Correcting for multiple testing using pFRR (Sect. 3.4), returns less than 1 expected number of false positives.

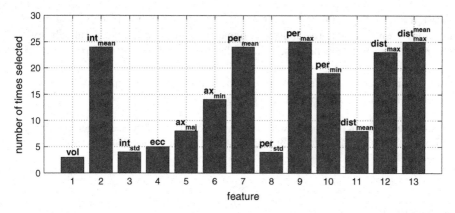

Fig. 4 The number of times a features was selected in the top (lowest RMSE) 25 multiple linear regression models is graphed. The y-axis shows the number of times the feature was selected and the x-axis is the feature selected. We can see that two features were selected in all the top 25 models, per_{max}, $dist_{max}^{mean}$, two were selected in 24 models, int_{mean}, per_{mean}, and one was selected in 23 models, $dist_{max}$. These five features are consistently selected which suggests their general importance in forming the model

Similar to Sect. 3.4, we also examine a more conservative selection of features by choosing those features that are consistently in the 25 models with lowest RMSE. We find that the features used in the lowest RMSE model and the features consistently chosen in the 25 lowest RMSE models *are the same*. These selected features are the ax_{maj} (chosen in 24 out of 25 models) and the per_{min} (chosen in 25 out of 25 models). We train another RF with 250 trees on $sel_{2RF} = \{ax_{maj}, per_{min}\}$ and show leave-one-out cross-validated results that outperform all our previous regression models, reported in Table 1 (row 6) and shown in Fig. 3b. This demonstrates that select novel morphological features, combined in a non-linear, non-parametric regression model can potentially provide more accurate predictions of MS physical disability than a linear model, and outperforms predictions based on spinal cord volume.

4 Conclusion

We proposed new morphological and appearance features to capture the subtle changes in a patient's spinal cord as it undergoes atrophy due to multiple sclerosis. These proposed features were combined in a regression model and our results indicate that they are potentially useful imaging biomarkers for multiple sclerosis. When only considering any one particular feature, the distance from the cord's center-of-mass to the cord's boundary, per_{min}, provided the strongest results and was an improvement over spinal cord volume at clinical prediction.

Our results also suggest that combining the selected features in a regression model improves the predictive ability over a simple linear regression model using any one of the tested features, including volume, alone. As well, a non-linear regression forest, trained on select morphological features, appears to be a promising approach to improve on the predictive ability of linear models. To ensure generalizability of our results (i.e. that the proposed biomarkers and models are not specific to our data and that our findings are not due to a Type I error), even though our data came from multiple centers, future work must involve larger datasets representing a greater variety in imaging, pathological, and clinical parameters.

Acknowledgments JK, RT, and GH were partially supported by NSERC and Biogen Idec Canada. CM was supported by the Canadian Breast Cancer Foundation and the Canadian Cancer Society Research Institute.

References

1. Benedetti, B., Rocca, M.A., Rovaris, M., Caputo, D., Zaffaroni, M., Capra, R., Bertolotto, A., Martinelli, V., Comi, G., Filippi, M.: A diffusion tensor MRI study of cervical cord damage in benign and secondary progressive multiple sclerosis patients. J. Neurol. Neurosurg, Psychiatry **81**(1), 26–30 (2010)
2. Criminisi, A., Shotton, J., Konukoglu, E.: Decision forests: a unified framework for classification, regression, density estimation, manifold learning and semi-supervised learning. Found. Trends Comput. Graph. Vision **7**(2–3), 81–227 (2011)
3. Fischer, J., Rudick, R., Cutter, G., Reingold, S.: The multiple sclerosis functional composite measure (MSFC): an integrated approach to MS clinical outcome assessment. Multiple Scler. **5**(4), 244–250 (1999)
4. Horsfield, M.A., Sala, S., Neema, M., Absinta, M., Bakshi, A., Sormani, M.P., Rocca, M.A., Bakshi, R., Filippi, M.: Rapid semi-automatic segmentation of the spinal cord from magnetic resonance images: application in multiple sclerosis. Neuroimage **50**(2), 446–455 (2010)
5. Kawahara, J., McIntosh, C., Tam, R., Hamarneh, G.: Globally optimal spinal cord segmentation using a minimal path in high dimensions. In: IEEE ISBI, pp. 836–839 (2013)
6. Kurtzke, J.F.: Rating neurologic impairment in multiple sclerosis an expanded disability status scale (EDSS). Neurology **33**(11), 1444–1452 (1983)
7. Lin, X., Tench, C., Turner, B., Blumhardt, L., Constantinescu, C.: Spinal cord atrophy and disability in multiple sclerosis over four years: application of a reproducible automated technique in monitoring disease progression in a cohort of the interferon β-1a (Rebif) treatment trial. J. Neurol. Neurosurg. Psychiatry **74**(8), 1090–1094 (2003)
8. Losseff, N., Webb, S., O'riordan, J., Page, R., Wang, L., Barker, G., Tofts, P., McDonald, W., Miller, D., Thompson, A.: Spinal cord atrophy and disability in multiple sclerosis a new reproducible and sensitive MRI method with potential to monitor disease progression. Brain **119**(3), 701–708 (1996)
9. Mann, R.S., Constantinescu, C.S., Tench, C.R.: Upper cervical spinal cord cross-sectional area in relapsing remitting multiple sclerosis: application of a new technique for measuring cross-sectional area on magnetic resonance images. J. Magn. Reson. Imaging **26**(1), 61–65 (2007)
10. McIntosh, C., Hamarneh, G.: Spinal crawlers: Deformable organisms for spinal cord segmentation and analysis. In: Larsen, R., Nielsen, M., Sporring, J. (eds.) MICCAI 2006, LNCS, vol. 4190, pp. 808–815. Springer, Heidelberg (2006)
11. McIntosh, C., Hamarneh, G., Toom, M., Tam, R.: Spinal cord segmentation for volume estimation in healthy and multiple sclerosis subjects using crawlers and minimal paths. In: IEEE HISB, pp. 25–31 (2011)

12. Rocca, M., Horsfield, M., Sala, S., Copetti, M., Valsasina, P., Mesaros, S., Martinelli, V., Caputo, D., Stosic-Opincal, T., Drulovic, J., Comi, G., Filippi, M.: A multicenter assessment of cervical cord atrophy among MS clinical phenotypes. Neurology **76**(24), 2096–2102 (2011)
13. Schnabel, J.A., Wang, L., Arridge, S.R.: Shape description of spinal cord atrophy in patients with MS. Comput. Assist. Radiol ICS **1124**, 286–291 (1996)
14. Storey, J.D.: A direct approach to false discovery rates. J. R. Stat. Soc. Ser. B (Stat. Method.) **64**(3), 479–498 (2002)
15. Tench, C.R., Morgan, P.S., Constantinescu, C.S.: Measurement of cervical spinal cord cross-sectional area by MRI using edge detection and partial volume correction. J. Magn. Reson. Imaging **21**(3), 197–203 (2005)
16. Valsasina, P., Rocca, M.A., Horsfield, M.A., Absinta, M., Messina, R., Caputo, D., Comi, G., Filippi, M.: Regional cervical cord atrophy and disability in multiple sclerosis: a voxel-based analysis. Radiology **266**(3), 853–861 (2013)

Classification of Spinal Deformities Using a Parametric Torsion Estimator

Jesse Shen, Stefan Parent and Samuel Kadoury

Abstract Adolescent idiopathic scoliosis (AIS) is a 3D deformity of the spine. However, the most widely accepted and used classification systems still rely on the 2D aspects of X-rays. Yet, a 3D classification of AIS remains elusive as there is no widely accepted 3D parameter in the clinical practice. The goal of this work is to propose a true 3D parameter that quantifies the torsion in thoracic AIS and automatically classifies patients in appropriate 3D sub-groups based on their diagnostic biplanar X-rays. First, an image-based approach anchored on prior statistical distributions is used to reconstruct the spine in 3D from biplanar X-rays. Geometric torsion measuring the twisting effect of the spine is then estimated using a novel technique that approximates local arc-lengths with parametric curve fitting at the neutral vertebra in the thoracolumbar/lumbar segment. We evaluated the method with a case series analysis of 255 patients with thoracic spine deformations recruited at our institution. The torsion index was evaluated in the thoracolumbar/lumbar junction in 3 sub-groups stratified by their lumbar modifier. An improvement in torsion estimation stability (mm^{-1}) was observed in comparison to a previous approach.

Supported by the CHU Sainte-Justine Academic Research Chair in Spinal Deformities, the Canada Research Chair in Medical Imaging and Assisted Interventions and the 3D committee of the Scoliosis Research Society.

J. Shen
CHU Sainte-Justine Research Center, Montréal, Canada
e-mail: jesse.shen@gmail.com

S. Parent
CHU Sainte-Justine Research Center, Department of Surgery, Université de Montréal,
Montréal, Canada
e-mail: stefan.parent@umontreal.ca

S. Kadoury (✉)
CHU Sainte-Justine Research Center, MEDICAL, École Polytechnique de Montréal,
Montréal, Canada
e-mail: samuel.kadoury@polymtl.ca

J. Yao et al. (eds.), *Computational Methods and Clinical Applications*
for Spine Imaging, Lecture Notes in Computational Vision and Biomechanics 17,
DOI: 10.1007/978-3-319-07269-2_7, © Springer International Publishing Switzerland 2014

An automatic classification based on torsion indices identified two groups: one with high torsion values ($2.81 \, \text{mm}^{-1}$) and one with low torsion values ($0.60 \, \text{mm}^{-1}$), showing the existence of two sub-groups of 3D deformations stemming from the same 2D class.

1 Introduction

Spinal deformity pathologies such as adolescent idiopathic scoliosis (AIS) are complex three-dimensional (3D) deformations of the trunk, described as a lateral deviation of the spine combined with asymmetric deformation of the vertebrae. Surgical treatment usually involves correction of the scoliotic curves with preshaped metal rods anchored in the vertebrae with screws and arthrodesis (bone fusion) of the intervertebral articulations. The most widely used classification paradigms for scoliosis are two-dimensional (2D) since they are based on spine X-rays in the sagittal and coronal planes. The Lenke classification [1] is one of the most accepted and widely used classification systems for AIS because it is easy to use and provides treatment recommendations. It offers a global evaluation of the scoliotic spine and offers better inter- as well as intra-observer reliability to previous systems [1–3]. However, it is still a 2D assessment of scoliosis that is based on the structurality and magnitude of Cobb angles in the proximal thoracic (PT), main thoracic (MT) as well as thoracolumbar/lumbar (TL/L) regions. Since 2D measurements and classification systems do not completely describe this 3D deformity, response to treatment for scoliosis can be at times difficult to accurately predict [4]. This is because 2D measurements are often measured on a plane of view that does not capture the position and orientation of the scoliosis curve in space. Consequently, two different scoliosis deformities may have similar 2D measurements. Applying similar treatments strategies based on similar 2D measurements may thus yield different surgical outcomes. Hence, there is a growing need to study scoliosis in 3D and develop 3D descriptors that will better characterize scoliosis and improve patient care.

Due to the 3D nature of AIS, the natural curvature properties of the spinal curve were also exploited with the goal of defining better indices to characterize the third dimension of scoliosis. Stokes et al. first introduced axial rotation (AR) as a local measure evaluated in the transverse plane to assess the effect of derotation maneuvers in surgical procedures [5]. Understanding how to classify and quantify 3D spinal deformities remains a difficult challenge in scoliosis. Recently, the Scoliosis Research Society (SRS) has recognized the need for 3D classification and mandated the 3D Scoliosis Committee to continue their efforts towards developing a 3D scheme for characterizing scoliosis. Duong et al. proposed an unsupervised fuzzy clustering technique in order to classify the 3D spine based on global shape descriptors [6]. Sangole et al. investigated the presence of subgroups within Lenke type-1 curves from 3D reconstructions of the spine, and proposed a new means to report 3D spinal deformities based on planes of maximal curvature (PMC) [7]. Recently, a multivariate analysis using manifold learning was able to identify four separate groups from the same cohort of thoracic deformities [8]. While these studies were able to identify different clusters of deformation using a series of 3D parameters, they were primarily qualitative and did not provide any quantifiable 3D measure to assess the severity of the deformation.

By using curved 3D line that passes through the thoracic and lumbar vertebra centroids to describe the general shape in the spine, several attempts have been made to measure the geometric torsion of the scoliotic curve. Geometric torsion is a property of a helicoidal line without specific relation to the rotation and deformation of the vertebrae themselve. Previous models demonstrated several limitations such as curve discontinuity caused by sequential modeling of the thoracic and lumbar segments or the inability to fit all types of scoliotic shapes. Therefore, geometric torsion was seldomly used as a reliable 3D geometric descriptor of scoliosis. To overcome this drawback, an approach was developed by Poncet et al. [9] to eliminate non-representative torsion spikes while minimizing the original geometric model deformity. This method was used to determine the amount of deviation (divergence) of the curved line from the plane determined by the tangent and normal vectors. These were then used to determine patterns of deformation based on torsion profiles. While the concept of scoliosis deformity was simplified using geometrical torsion by proposing a series of classification patterns, the method presented by Poncet et al. showed some limitations with respect to high sensitivity of inaccuracies in the 3D reconstruction, affecting the interpolated curvilinear shape of the spine. Furthermore, this measurement can only provide a local index at the vertebral level without a global measurement for an entire spinal segment. To circumvent these limitations, an alternative scheme for estimating curvature and torsion of planar and spatial curves was proposed, based on weighted least-square fitting and local arc-length approximation [10]. The method is simple enough to admit a convergence analysis that takes into account the effect of noise or inaccuracies in the 3D modeling of the spine.

In this paper, we propose a framework that infers the true 3D torsion parameter in AIS from biplanar X-rays images and automatically classifies patients in appropriate 3D sub-groups based on their torsion values. The general approach is described as follows. We first use a personalized 3D spine shape reconstructed from biplanar X-rays to obtain a landmark-based representation of the patient's thoracic and lumbar spine. The spine is divided into three anatomical regions based on the spinal curve's second derivatives. Geometric torsion measuring the twisting effect of the spine is then estimated at the junction of the segmental curves, using a novel technique by approximating local arc-lengths at the neutral vertebra in the thoracolumbar/lumbar segment. The torsion indices are then sent to a c-means classifier to identify the correct 3D sub-group. One of the applications is to help surgeons treat complicated deformity cases by offering a reliable predictor of the 3D deformation from the preoperative models and adapt the surgical strategy based on the defamation class. Section 2 presents the method in terms of geometric modeling and torsion estimator. Experiments are showed in Sect. 3, with a discussion in Sect. 4 and a conclusion in Sect. 5.

2 Methods

We now explain in more detail the components of the framework. First, we detail the statistical and image-based biplanar reconstruction method, which is performed on biplanar X-rays taken at baseline or follow-up prior to surgery. The model is then used to estimate the parametric torsion index at the transition zones (e.g. at the junction of the thoracic and lumbar segments). Finally, the torsion estimator is used to classify patients and identify different subgroups from the studied population.

2.1 Training Data

The statistical model used for the initial 3D reconstruction is built from a dataset of 711 spine models, demonstrating several types of deformities. Each scoliotic spine in the database was obtained from biplanar stereo-reconstructions. It is modeled with 12 thoracic and 5 lumbar vertebrae (17 in total), represented by 6 landmarks on each vertebra (4 pedicle extremities and 2 endplate center points), which were annotated by a radiologist. Segmentation of the scoliotic vertebrae on the X-ray images was performed by using generic vertebra priors obtained from serial CT-scan reconstructions of a cadaver specimen. Models were segmented using a connecting cube algorithm [11] with 1-mm-thick CT-scan slices taken at 1-mm steps throughout the dry spine. The atlas is composed of 17 cadaver vertebrae (12 thoracic and 5 lumbar). The same 6 precise anatomical landmarks (4 pedicle tips and 2 on the vertebral body) were annotated on each individual model.

2.2 Personalized 3D Spine Reconstruction

From calibrated coronal and sagittal X-ray images $I_{i=\{1,2\}}$ of the patient's spine, a personalized 3D model is obtained by means of a reconstruction method merging statistical and image-based models based on our previous work [12], and summarized in Fig. 1. The approximate 3D spine centerline $\mathbf{r}_i(t)$, obtained from quadratic curves extracted from the images is first embedded onto the 3D database of scoliotic spines (M) to predict an initial spine, modeled by 17: (N) vertebrae (12 thoracic, 5 lumbar), 6 points per vertebra (4 pedicle tips and 2 endplate midpoints). To map the high-dimensional 3D curve $\mathbf{r}$ assumed to lie on a non-linear manifold into a low-dimensional subspace, we first determine the manifold reconstruction weights W to reconstruct point i from it's K neighbors, and then determine the global internal coordinates of Y by solving $\Phi(Y) = \sum_{i=1}^{M} \| Y_i - \sum_{j=1}^{K} W_{ij} Y_j \|^2$.

The projection point Y_{new} is used to generate an appropriately scaled model from an analytical method based on nonlinear regression using a Radial Basis Function kernel function f, with D is the dimensionality of the spine and X_{preop} to perform the inverse mapping such that $X_{\text{preop}} = [f_1(Y_{\text{new}}), ..., f_D(Y_{\text{new}})]$ with $X_{\text{preop}} =$

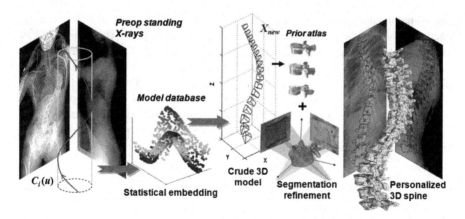

Fig. 1 Personalized spine 3D reconstruction from pre-operative biplanar X-rays [12]

$(s_1, s_2, \ldots, s_{17})$, where s_i is a vertebra model defined by $s_i = (p_1, p_2, \ldots, p_6)$, and $p_i \in \mathfrak{R}^3$ is a 3D vertebral landmark.

This crude statistical 3D model is refined with an individual scoliotic vertebra segmentation approach by extending 2D geodesic active regions in 3D, in order to evolve prior deformable 3D surfaces by level sets optimization. An atlas of vertebral meshes $S_i = \{x_{i1}, \ldots, x_{iN}\}$ with triangles x_j are initially positioned and oriented from their respective 6 precise landmarks p_i. The surface evolution is then regulated by the gradient map and image intensity distributions [13], where $E_{RAG} = \alpha E_{CAG}(S) + (1 - \alpha)E_R(S)$ is the energy function with the edge and region-based components controlled by α determined empirically, are defined as:

$$E_{CAG} = \sum_{i=1}^{2} \oint_{S_i} \frac{1}{1 + |\nabla I_i(u_i)|^\alpha} d u_i \; ; \; E_R = -\sum_{i=1}^{2} \iint_{\Pi_i(S_i)} \log(p_R(I_i(u_i))) d u_i \quad (1)$$

with Π_i as the perspective projection parameters, and p_R is a Gaussian distribution. The projected silhouettes of the morphed 3D models would therefore match the 2D information on the biplanar X-rays in the image domain u, replicating the specifics of a particular scoliotic deformity. At the end of process, the 3D landmark coordinates p_i and corresponding polygonal vertebral meshes S_i are optimal with regards to statistical distribution and image correspondences.

2.3 Parametric Torsion Estimator

Torsion definition: Once the personalized 3D spine model is obtained, we use a torsion estimation method based on weighted least-squares fitting of vertebra centroids, approximating the samples by a parametric curve that have one of its coordinate functions given by a second (or third)-order polynomial [10]. The estimator has been shown to converge under reasonable conditions over the sampling of the curve and the amplitude of the noise. Here, the tangent vector for the parameterized spinal curve $\mathbf{r}(s)$ is defined by $\mathbf{T}(s) = \mathbf{r}'(s)$. The normal vector is defined by $\mathbf{N}(s) = \mathbf{r}''(s)/\|\mathbf{r}''(s)\|$, and the bi-normal vector is given by the cross-product of $\mathbf{T}(s)$ and $\mathbf{N}(s)$, i.e., $\mathbf{B}(s) = \mathbf{T}(s) \times \mathbf{N}(s)$. Using these definitions, the torsion is defined by the formula $\mathbf{B}'(s) = \tau(s)\mathbf{N}(s)$. When the curve $\mathbf{r}(t)$ is not parameterized by the arc-length, the torsion is given by:

$$\tau(t) = -\frac{(\mathbf{r}' \times \mathbf{r}'') \cdot \mathbf{r}'''}{\|\mathbf{r}' \times \mathbf{r}''\|^2} \tag{2}$$

Torsion estimator using weighted least-squares fitting: If we consider the landmarks p_i of the personalized 3D model, i.e., a finite sequence of sample points of $\mathbf{r}$, perturbed by a random noise (reconstruction errors), assuming the spinal curve to be parameterized by the arc-length, the torsion estimation needs an approximation of the first, second, and third derivatives of $\mathbf{r}(s)$.

Previous studies have shown that the torsion phenomena is predominantly present at neutral vertebrae of the scoliotic spine, which represent the transition point between segmental regions at the thoracolumbar/lumbar junction [9]. If we consider the point $\mathbf{p}_0$ to be a neutral vertebra, the estimation of the derivatives of $\mathbf{r}$ at $\mathbf{p}_0$ will be performed from a window of $2q + 1$ points around $\mathbf{p}_0 : \{\mathbf{p}_{-q}, \mathbf{p}_{-q+1}, \cdots, \mathbf{p}_q\}$, such that $-q$ represents the upper apical vertebra, and $+q$ is the lower apical vertebra. These are determined automatically by analyzing the output model S and identifying the anatomical regions where the spinal curve's second derivatives are zero. Apical vertebrae represent the most deviated vertebrae form the central sacral vertical line for each of these regions.

The noise at a point $\mathbf{p}_i$ is modelled by a random vector η_i, normal to $\mathbf{r}$ at $\mathbf{p}_i$, and the random variables η_i are assumed to be independent and identically distributed (i.i.d.), with zero mean and variance σ^2 as shown in Fig. 2a. Let s_i be the arc-length corresponding to the sample $\mathbf{p}_i$. The estimates of $\mathbf{r}'(0)$, $\mathbf{r}''(0)$ and $\mathbf{r}'''(0)$ are obtained by a weighted least-squares minimization. The weight w_i of point $\mathbf{p}_i$ must be positive, relatively large for small $\|s_i\|$ and relatively small for large $\|s_i\|$. For example, one can consider weights of the form $w_i = \alpha \exp(-\beta s_i^2)/s_i^k$, or simply $w_i = 1$. For spatial curves, the torsion estimator fits a cubic parametric curve to the sample points. Assuming that $\mathbf{p}_0 = \mathbf{r}(0) = (0, 0, 0)$, x_0', x_0'' and x_0''' should minimize:

$$E_x(x_0', x_0'', x_0''') = \sum_{i=-q}^{q} w_i \left(x_i - (x_0's_i + \frac{1}{2}x_0''s_i^2 + \frac{1}{6}x_0'''s_i^3) \right)^2. \tag{3}$$

Considering we can again use an approximation of s_i, the above equation can be solved by matrix inversion [10]. A similar approach is used to compute

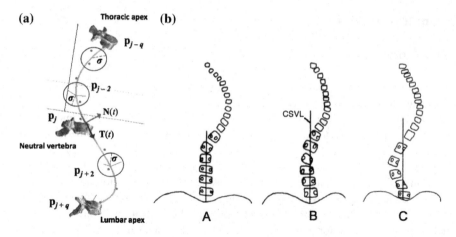

Fig. 2 **a** Torsion estimator model using a sampled curve with noise. **b** Lenke type-1 examples with lumbar modifiers (A, B, C) from the central sacral vertical line (*CSVL*)

y_0', y_0'', y_0''', z_0', z_0'' and z_0''', using an independent coordinates method which estimates the derivatives in each dimension. Using the above derivatives estimates, Eq. (2) gives the parametric torsion.

Clustering algorithm: A fuzzy c-means clustering technique is then used in order to group patients with similar torsion values together, while keeping the mean torsion of each group as distinct as possible. This *soft* clustering algorithm allows for patient torsion values to be classified in multiple groups, while providing the different degrees of confidence for belonging to the various group. This means that each patient torsion value does not need to belong to a particular group, but may belong more strongly to one group in particular.

2.4 Analysis Methodology

An inter- and intra-group statistical analysis was performed to assess torsion values and how they relate to other 2D, as well as 3D spinal parameters such as the orientation of the PMC in each regional curve, measuring the orientation of the plane where the projected Cobb angle is maximum, to the sagittal plane. We also measure Cobb angles in the MT and TL/L segments. Kyphosis, defined by the angle between T2 and T12 on the sagittal plane, as well as lordosis (angle between L1 and S1) were finally evaluated to find differences in Lenke type-1A, Lenke type-1B and Lenke type-1C (Fig. 2b). For each case, torsion was estimated with both the proposed method and with the approach by Poncet et al. [9]. An ANOVA test with Bonferonni correction was applied in order to evaluate differences between the cluster groups.

3 Clinical Validation

3.1 Clinical Data

A cohort of 255 patients diagnosed with adolescent idiopathic scoliosis (AIS) recruited at our institution was used for this preliminary study. The inclusion criteria was patients classified as having a Lenke type-1 deformity [1]. A 3D spinal reconstruction, generating vertebral landmarks p_i on each vertebra, was obtained for each case. The mean thoracic Cobb angle for this cohort was $51.4 \pm 13.85°$ and lumbar mean Cobb angle of $35.5 \pm 13.21°$. The Lenke classification was confirmed by an expert in scoliosis research at our institution, using the biplanar radiographs available for each patient. Patients with any pathology other than AIS were excluded for the study. All patients classified as having a Lenke type-1 deformity with rare conditions such as left thoracic deformities were also excluded in this study. Each eligible patient was assigned a lumbar spine modifier (A, B, C). In all, this study includes 209 Lenke type-1A, 31 Lenke type-1B and 15 Lenke type-1C deformities were included.

3.2 Torsion Estimation in Scoliotic Spines

As it was shown in numerous studies, normal spines lies in a single plane (sagittal), and thus, according to the definition, have no torsion. In reality, the ideal spine does not exist, but values of parametric torsion in the control group of normal patients ($N = 5$) were small. In all cases, the maximum absolute values of torsion were found to be $<0.08 \, mm^{-1}$. In the scoliotic group, maximum values of torsion ranged from 0.15 to $5.63 \, mm^{-1}$. Geometric torsion in normal spines is much less than that in scoliotic spines.

The torsion values of the 209 patients with Lenke type 1A, 31 patients with Lenke type 1B and 15 patients with Lenke type 1C were evaluated, which takes $0.8 \, s$ on average per case to compute. Figure 3 presents these results in comparison to a previous torsion estimation approach [9]. Using the proposed approach, a statistically significant difference ($p = 0.002$) between the torsion values of Lenke type-1A and Lenke type-1C cases was observed, while no statistically significant differences were found between either groups using [9]. Furthermore, the parametric torsion estimator offers more stable and reproducible values, demonstrating lower standard deviation values compared to [9] which finds no pattern between groups 1A, 1B and 1C.

3.3 Automatic Classification Results

The fuzzy c-means clustering algorithm was performed on the 255 patients and identified two groups of torsion values: one group with higher torsion value means of $2.81 \, mm^{-1}$ ($N = 48$) and one group with lower torsion value means of 0.60 mm^{-1} ($N = 207$) respectively. Figures 4 and 5 illustrate sample cases for both groups. Table 1 presents the characteristics for both groups. Results first show that

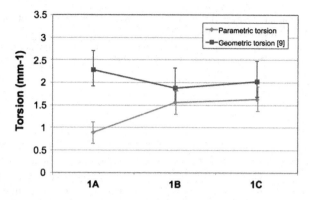

Fig. 3 Mean and standard deviation torsion values with respect to lumbar modifier classes, in comparison to a previous torsion estimation approach by [9]

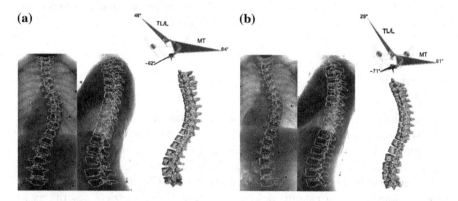

Fig. 4 Sample low torsion cases, with resulting 3D reconstructed models and axial view with corresponding PMCs. **a** Torsion value at TL/L junction of 0.46 mm^{-1}. **b** Torsion value at TL/L junction of 0.63 mm^{-1}

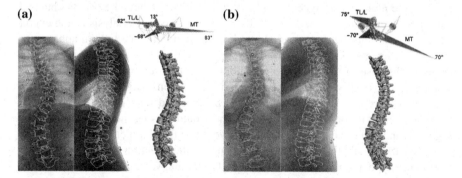

Fig. 5 Sample high torsion cases, with resulting 3D reconstructed models and axial view with corresponding PMCs. **a** Torsion value at TL/L junction of 2.83 mm^{-1}. **b** Torsion value at TL/L junction of 3.75 mm^{-1}

Table 1 Composition and characteristics (mean torsion, standard deviation) of the two torsion clusters determined by the c-means classification

	N	% A	% B	% C	Mean	S.D.	Maximum	Minimum
Cluster 1	207	86.1	9.6	4.3	0.60	0.41	1.64	0.05
Cluster 2	48	64.6	22.9	12.5	2.81	0.77	5.06	1.70

while 1A deformations are predominant in both clusters due the larger sample size ($N = 207$), the high torsion cluster is composed with a greater portion of cases with 1B and 1C modifiers. This indicates how higher torsion is linked to the curvature in the lumbar region. This is confirmed with the difference in thoracolumbar/lumbar PMC angulation between the high torsion group (56.4°) and the low torsion group (49.2°), which is statistically significant ($p = 0.030$). Also, a statistically significant difference ($p = 0.014$) in main thoracic PMC angulation was found between the high torsion group (79.8°) and the low torsion group (73.7°).

4 Discussion

With the intent of determining optimal surgical strategies and treatments for patients with AIS, quantification and classification of spinal deformities such as AIS in 3D remains challenging because of the difficulty of translating complex geometrical concepts into clinically applicable paradigms. Recent studies have investigated into pattern classification based on explicit parameters. Classification systems have therefore emerged from patterns detected on these 3D geometrical descriptors to discriminate various types of spine deformities.

Our results show an increase in torsion values as a function of the lumbar spine modifier as Lenke type-1A were shown to have the lowest torsion value means and type-1C the highest with type-1B in between. This contradicts the results obtained with a previous torsion estimator based on a local derivative analysis of the curve, which finds no link between torsion and lumbar modifiers. While both approaches show high deviations due to the intra-group variability, this deviation is of lesser extent in the case of the proposed method. Our results confirm the findings of [7] that spinal curves in scoliosis have abnormal orientations in 3D space with respect to the sagittal plane. The results shown can be expected since type-1A deformities would represent no or little lumbar curve and would thus be more aligned with its sagittal plane while the type-1C deformity would be the complete opposite. Thus, a thoracic curve would thus have a greater change in the direction with Lenke type-1C than Lenke type-1A and will thus have a higher torsion value.

The ability of torsion to differentiate new subgroups with Lenke type-1 deformities is emphasized when clustering the entire cohort into two groups. The high torsion group was found to have a greater percentage of Lenke 1B and 1C patients compared to the low torsion group, which was primarily composed on Lenke 1A patients. This is confirmed with the orientation of the thoracolumbar/lumbar PMC plane, which was more deviated towards the coronal plane in the high torsion group as shown in Figs. 4 and 5. This effect was also observed in the thoracic PMC. Patients with high torsion values tend to have two PMCs that are highly angulated with respect to each other. Conceptually, this means that a deformity with highly angulated PMCs will have a greater torsion values since the amplitude of the change of curve orientation is greater in this situation.

The technique presented in this paper provides a mean to evaluate the flexibility of the spine in the thoracolumbar region, which is critical to determine the optimal surgical strategy and fusion levels. Populations of 3D scoliotic patients obtained from a hybrid statistical and image-based approach from 2D projections can be analyzed and subsequently classified in order to determine patterns in pathological cases. Hence personalized 3D reconstructions of thoracic (T)/lumbar (L) spines obtained from a cohort of Lenke Type-1 patients were analyzed with a torsion estimator algorithm by approximating local arc-lengths at the neutral vertebra in the thoracolumbar/lumbar segment.

5 Conclusion and Future Work

We presented a method for quantifying geometric torsion of 3D reconstructed spine models from biplanar X-ray images. By taking a more global approach for torsion estimation, using parametric curve fitting that minimizes the effects of noisy data, the proposed methodology yields torsion values that are more reliable to the actual twisting effect in the scoliotic spine. This allows for a quantitative analysis of the spinal deformity based on the numerical values of geometric torsion that is more representative of the true torsion phenomena. The results of our current study suggest that a more stable estimation of the 3D torsion effect at transition zones in scoliosis is within reach. The advantage of using numerical values to classify scoliosis is that it simplifies the work needed for the observer and reduces the classification variability between them. Thus, by proposing geometric torsion as a numerical 3D index for a quantifiable analysis of scoliosis, this opens the possibility for a 3D classification paradigm of scoliosis that will not only be more user friendly, but also more accurate in describing this deformity. Future work will look at extending this analysis to other types of classes, such as double thoracic and lumbar deformations.

References

1. Lenke, L., Betz, R., Harms, J., et al.: Adolescent idiopathic scoliosis: a new classification to determine extent of spinal arthrodesis. J. Bone Joint Surg. **83**, 1169–1181 (2001)
2. King, H., Moe, J., Bradford, D., et al.: The selection of fusion levels in thoracic idiopathic scoliosis. J. Bone Joint Surg. Am. **65**, 1302–1313 (1983)
3. Ogon, M., Giesinger, K., Behensky, H., et al.: Interobserver and intraobserver reliability of Lenke's new scoliosis classication system. Spine **27**, 858–862 (2002)

4. Stokes, I.: Three-dimensional terminology of spinal deformity: a report presented to the Scoliosis Research Society by the Scoliosis Research Society Working Group on 3D Terminology of Spinal Deformity. Spine **19**, 236–248 (1994)

5. Stokes, I., Bigalow, L., Moreland, M.: Three-dimensional spinal curvature in idiopathic scoliosis. J. Orthop. Res. **5**, 102–113 (1987)

6. Duong, L., Cheriet, F., Labelle, H.: Three-dimensional classification of spinal deformities using fuzzy clustering. Spine **31**, 923–930 (2006)

7. Sangole, A., Aubin, C., Labelle, H., et al.: Three-Dimensional classification of thoracic scoliotic curves. Spine **34**, 91–99 (2009)

8. Kadoury, S., Labelle, H.: Classification of three-dimensional thoracic deformities in adolescent idiopathic scoliosis from a multivariate analysis. Eur. Spine J. **21**, 40–49 (2012)

9. Poncet, P., Dansereau, J., Labelle, H.: Geometric torsion in idiopathic Scoliosis: three-dimensional analysis and proposal for a new classification. Spine **26**, 2235–2243 (2001)

10. Lewiner, T., Gomes Jr, J., Lopes, H., et al.: Curvature and torsion estimators based on parametric curve fitting. Comput. Graph. **29**, 641–655 (2005)

11. Lorensen, W., Cline, H.: Marching cubes: a high resolution 3-D surface construction algorithm. Comput. Graph. **4**, 163–169 (1988)

12. Kadoury, S., Cheriet, F., Labelle, H.: Personalized X-ray 3D reconstruction of the scoliotic spine from statistical and image-based models. IEEE Trans. Med. Imaging **28**, 1422–1435 (2009)

13. Paragios, N., Deriche, R.: Geodesic active regions: new paradigm to deal with frame partition problems in CV. Vis. Comm. Image Repre. **13**, 249–268 (2002)

Lumbar Spine Disc Herniation Diagnosis with a Joint Shape Model

Raja S. Alomari, Jason J. Corso, Vipin Chaudhary
and Gurmeet Dhillon

Abstract Lower Back Pain (LBP) is the second most common neurological ailment in the United States after the headache. It costs over $100 billion annually in treatment and related rehabilitation costs including worker compensation. In fact, it is the most common reason for lost wages and missed work days. Degenerative Disc Disease (DDD) is the major abnormality that causes LBP. Moreover, Magnetic Resonance Imaging (MRI) test is the main clinically approved non-invasive imaging modality for the diagnosis of DDD. However, there is over 50 % inter- and intra-observer variability in the MRI interpretation that urges the need for standardized mechanisms in MRI interpretation. In this chapter, we propose a Computer Aided Diagnosis (CAD) System for Disc Degenerative Disease detection from clinical Magnetic Resonance Imaging (MRI). This CAD produces a reproducible and clinically accurate diagnosis of the DDD for lumbar spine. We design a classifier to automatically detect degenerated disc (also clinically known as Herniation) using shape potentials. We extract these shape potentials by jointly applying an active shape model (ASM) and a gradient vector flow snake model (GVF-snake). The ASM roughly segments the disc by the detection of a certain point distribution around the disc. Then, we use this point distribution to initialize a GVF-snake model to delineate the posterior disc segment. We then extract the set of shape potentials for our Gibbs-based classifier. The whole work flow is fully automated given the full clinical MRI. We validate our model on

R. S. Alomari · J. J. Corso · V. Chaudhary (✉)
State University of New York (SUNY) at Buffalo, Buffalo, NY, USA
e-mail: vipin@buffalo.edu

R. S. Alomari
The University of Jordan, Amman, Jordan
e-mail: ralomari@buffalo.edu

J. J. Corso
e-mail: jcorso@buffalo.edu

G. Dhillon
Proscan Radiology Buffalo, Buffalo, NY, USA
e-mail: gdhillon@proscan.com

J. Yao et al. (eds.), *Computational Methods and Clinical Applications*
for Spine Imaging, Lecture Notes in Computational Vision and Biomechanics 17,
DOI: 10.1007/978-3-319-07269-2_8, © Springer International Publishing Switzerland 2014

65 clinical MRI cases (6 discs each) and achieve an average of 93.9 % classification accuracy. Our shape-based classifier is superior in classification accuracy compared to the state-of-the-art work on this problem that reports 86 and 91 % on 34 and 33 cases, respectively.

1 Introduction

Low Back Pain has a major economic impact in the United States with over $100 billion annually in related treatment and rehabilitation costs [1]. It is the most common reason why patients visit a physician office besides the common cold. In fact, it is the most common reason patients visited the emergency room in the U.S. in 2008. There were over 3.4 million emergency rooms visits, an average of 9400 visits a day, specifically for Low Back Pain [2]. Low back Pain has high societal impact as it disrupts individuals lives impacting over 80 % of people [3]. Moreover, it is the most common reason behind job-related disability and is the second most common neurological ailment after headache [3]. It is a prominent chronic disease that causes major disruption in people's lives.

Nevertheless, the diagnostic decision is highly subjective and relies on two major factors: the radiologist's diagnostic report and the neurological exam findings. The most common current clinically approved standard for Low Back Pain diagnosis is the Magnetic Resonance Imaging (MRI) procedure. However, individual radiologists interpreting clinical Magnetic Resonance Imaging (MRI) studies are highly subjective with over 50 % inter-observer variation [4]. This high inter-radiologist variation significantly influences therapeutic treatment, medical insurance decision makers, and judiciary personnel decisions. On the other hand, the clinical diagnosis is highly variable that nothing certain can be said regarding the clinical diagnosis of Low Back Pain [5]. Providing a reproducible computerized MRI interpretation may reduce the existing variability, and hence, standardize the diagnostic decisions that lead to reduced costs on unnecessary treatment. Surprisingly, there is no CAD system for the lumbar spine that yet has clinical applicability. We are building our system motivated by the clinical practice of lumbar diagnosis. In this chapter, we propose a reliable, robust, and accurate diagnosis for disc herniation which is the main condition that causes failed low back syndrome. We, however, point out that the nomenclature has been a controversial issue in spine diseases which is outside the scope of this chapter. We target the problem of the leak of the nucleus pulposus (as shown in Fig. 1) that causes pressure on the nerve root resulting in the pain and numbness to the patient where the pain, most of the time, irritates to the knees causing major disruption of the patients life. We use the nomenclature of Fardon et al. [7] that has been endorsed by the major American and European radiologists associations including ASSR, ASNR, AANS, CNS, ESNR, and many others. For the rest of this chapter, we call this condition as Herniation.

Disc herniation always occurs in the posterior segment of the disc. The inner gel-like material of the disc, nucleus pulposus, leaks out pressing on a nerve root through a tear in the fibrous wall of the disc, annulus fibrosus [8], as illustrated in

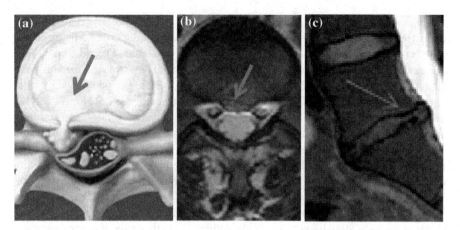

Fig. 1 **a** A right-sided disc herniation illustrative model [6]. **b** Axial view (*bottom-up*) MRI of a right-sided disc herniation from our data. **c** Corresponding sagittal view of the herniated disc from our dataset

Fig. 1, where we show an axial illustrative model and a corresponding clinical MRI (from our dataset) for a right-sided disc herniation with both the axial and sagittal views.

Shape of the posterior segment of the disc, from the sagittal view, is the primary diagnostic tool for the radiologist. The axial view is used for confirmation and for quantification. Working in the sagittal view, our method extracts information of the posterior segment of the disc in a two-step process. First, we use an active shape model to roughly localize a point distribution for the disc body. Then, we have a GVF-snake to delineate the posterior segment of the disc using the outcome of the ASM as its initialization. Because the ASM is a linear model and captures Gaussian point distributions, we add the GVF-snake step to delineate the non-linear shape of the disc posterior segment which is the main technical innovation in this chapter. We validate our method on a clinical dataset of sixty-five cases and achieve over 93 % average classification accuracy.

We also compare our results to the most recent work on disc herniation diagnosis by Alomari et al. [9, 10] that jointly model shape and intensity and we substantially outperform their results. Moreover, our shape-based classifier outperforms the recent work of Michopoulou et al. [11] which is based on an intensity-based classifier. Both recent works test on 33 and 34 cases with an average herniation detection accuracy of 91 and 88 %, respectively. We validate our model on substantially variable dataset of 65 cases and achieve better accuracy over 93 %. Many researchers have proposed methods for the diagnosis of certain vertebral column abnormalities. Bounds et al. [12] utilized a neural network for the diagnosis of back pain and sciatica. Sciatica might be caused by lumbar disc Herniation as well as many other reasons. They have three groups of doctors to perform diagnosis as their validation mechanism. They claimed a better accuracy than the doctors in the diagnosis. However, the lack of data prohibited them from full validation of their system. Similarly, Vaughn [13] conducted a research study on using neural network for assisting orthopedic surgeons in the diagnosis of lower back pain. They classified LBP into three broad clinical categories: Simple Low Back Pain (SLBP), Root Pain (ROOTP), and Abnormal Illness Behavior (AIB) and about 200 cases were collected over the period of 2 years with diagnosis from radiologists. They used 25 features to train the Neural Network (NN) including symptoms clinical assessment results. The NN achieved 99 % of training accuracy and 78.5 % of testing accuracy. This clearly shows training data overfitting.

Tsai et al. [14] used geometrical features (shape, size and location) to diagnose herniation from 3D MRI and CT axial (transverse sections) volumes of the discs. In contrast, we do not presume the availability of the full volume axial view as it is not a clinical standard. They patented their work as a visualization tool for educational purposes. Recently, Michopoulou et al. [11] applied three variations of fuzzy c-means (FCM) to perform atlas-based disc segmentation. Then, they used this segmentation for classification of the disc as either a normal or degenerative disc. They used an intensity-based Bayesian classifier and achieved 86–88 % classification accuracy on 34 cases (five discs each) based on their semi-automatic segmentation of the disc. Similarly, Alomari et al. [9, 10] proposed utilizing a shape and an intensity-based classifier that utilizes an active shape model to extract the shape potentials. However, because the ASM cannot capture the non-linearly shaped posterior segment of the herniated disc, they achieved about 91 % on 33 clinical cases. We extend both these works and present our technical novelty by concentrating on the posterior segment of the disc and capturing that with an additional GVF-snake model on top of the ASM. Furthermore, we reduce the effect of intensity-based information due to the signal intensity inhomogeneity with clinical MRI. We also significantly add variability in the dataset by validating our joint model on 65 clinical cases as opposed to 33 and 34 cases. Furthermore, we achieved an average of 93 % accuracy which substantially outperforms both state-of-the-art results given the dataset size difference.

2 Proposed Method

Our approach has four steps: Disc Localization, Disc Segmentation, Herniation Delineation, and Herniation Classification. This section explains each step:

Disc Localization: The system automatically locates the middle sagittal slice from the MRI volume by index. Then our automatic method starts by a localization step that provides a point inside each disc using the two-level probabilistic model proposed by Corso et al. [15, 16]. Their model labels the set of discs with high level labels $D = \{d_1, d_2, \ldots, d_6\}$ where each $d_i = (x_i, y_i)^{\mathsf{T}}$ is the coordinates of the disc point (some point in the disc). They solve the optimization problem:

$$D^* = \arg \max_{D} \sum_{L} P(L, D|I) = \arg \max_{D} \sum_{L} P(L|D, I) P(D) \tag{1}$$

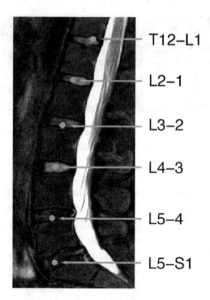

Fig. 2 Labeling lumbar discs in a sagittal T2-weighted MRI [15, 16]

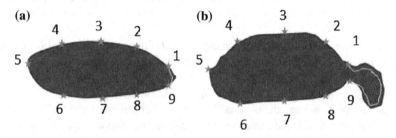

Fig. 3 Illustrative model (sagittal view) for **a** clinically normal disc **b** herniated disc showing the point distribution ($k_1 - k_9$) as well as a contour (*yellow*) that delineates the edge map between points k_1 and k_9. This figure shows the *irregular shape* of the normal disc

where $L = \{l_i, \forall i \in L\}$ is a set of auxiliary variables, called disc-label variables that are introduced to infer D from the sagittal image. Each disc-label variable can take a value of $\{-1, +1\}$ for non-disc or disc, respectively. The disc-labels make it plausible to separate the disc variables from the image intensities, i.e., the disc-label L variables capture the local pixel-level intensity models while the disc variables D capture the high-level geometric and contextual models of the full set of discs. The optimization is solved with a generalized expectation minimization (gEM) algorithm [15, 16]. Figure 2 shows a lumbar sagittal view with labeled discs. Then we obtain a fixed window of 60 × 120 pixels around each point. This sub-image size is enough to provide the whole disc region for each of the discs connected to the five lumbar vertebrae as shown in Fig. 2.

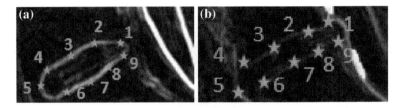

Fig. 4 Feature image result of the range filter R for **a** Normal disc. **b** Herniated disc. The ASM point distribution is shown according to the map in Fig. 3

Disc Segmentation: We use an active shape model [17] for roughly segmenting the disc body boundary. This step finds the rough shape of the disc body regardless of the herniated (posterior) part. To prepare the training data, we manually select the image slice where herniation is most obvious. Then, we manually mark nine landmark points according to the map shown in Fig. 3. Specifying these landmarks locations is only based on our expertise in the disc segmentation. We name these landmark points from k_1 to k_9. Similar to [17], we initially calculate the mean shape $\bar{x} = \frac{1}{N} \sum_1^N x$ where N is the size of the training data. Then each disc shape x_i, where $i \in \{1, \ldots, N\}$, is recursively aligned to the mean shape $\bar{x}$ using generalized Procrustes Analysis to remove translational, rotational, and isotropic scaling from the shape.

Then, we model the remaining variance around the mean shape with principal components analysis (PCA) to extract the eigenvectors of the covariance matrix associated with 98 % of the remaining point position variance according to the standard method for deriving the ASM's linear shape representation.

However, we do not use the original MRI image for training the ASM. Rather, we utilize a feature image I that enhances the disc shape by emphasizing the boundaries of the disc and the Thecal Sac (the extension of the spinal canal at the lumbar level [8]). We produce I by applying a range filter R on the pixel-wise addition of the normalized co-registered T1- and T2-weighted protocols of the sagittal images $I = R(T1 + T2)$ where T1 and T2 are the normalized T1- and T2-weighted MRI images for the same case. These two images are manually co-registered during the acquisition of the MRI in the clinical standard. R is the range filter operator where the intensity levels in each 3×3 window are replaced by the range value (maximum - minimum) in that window. This operator R has high values in abrupt-change regions and small values in smooth regions. Figure 4 shows the features images I for a normal- and a herniated-disc. The ASM landmark points are also shown in the figure to clarify the ASM land-marking step.

To apply ASM for detection of the point distribution of the disc body boundary, we apply the mean shape $\bar{x}$ around the disc point produced by the localization step. Then, we allow the ASM to converge and obtain the boundary.

We apply the GVF-snake by initializing its contour (to the line connecting the two points k_1 and k_9). Figure 5 show two examples of the convergence of the GVF-snake for both a normal disc (Fig. 5a) and a herniated one (Fig. 5b). The figure also shows

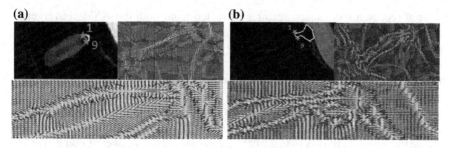

Fig. 5 (*Top-left*) Shows the resulting GVF-contour for **a** normal **b** abnormal, on T2-weighted image. (*Top-right*) The corresponding normalized GVF field showing the two initialization landmarks k_1 and k_9. (*Bottom*) A zoomed version of the GVF field to clearly show the vectors

the normalized gradient vector field for the sub-image as well as a zoomed GVF field for the area of interest (posterior part of the disc).

Herniation Delineation: The ASM segmentation of the disc cannot capture the inherent variations produced by the disc herniation at the posterior segment of the disc. Furthermore, we seek for a single model for the disc regardless whether it is herniated or not. Thus, we use an active contour to delineate the posterior segment of the disc. We select the GVF-snake proposed by Xu and Prince [18] because it has been proved to move toward desired image properties such as edges including concavities. GVF-snake is the parametric curve that solves:

$$\mathbf{x}_t(s, t) = \alpha \mathbf{x}''(s, t) - \beta \mathbf{x}''''(s, t) + \mathbf{v} \tag{2}$$

where α and β are weighting parameters that control the contour's tension and rigidity, respectively. x'' and x'''' are the second and fourth derivatives, respectively, of x. $\mathbf{v}(x, y)$ is the gradient vector flow (GVF), $s \in [0, 1]$, and t is time component to make a dynamic snake curve from $x(s)$ yielding $x(s, t)$.

GVF-snake requires an edge map that is a binary image highlighting the desired features (edges) of the image. Most researchers use Canny edge detector or Sobel operator on the original image such as [19] for liver segmentation. We present the GVF-snake with a canny edge map applied on our feature image $\mathcal{I}$.

Herniation Classification: We design a binary Bayesian classifier:

$$n^* = \arg\max_n P(n|\mathsf{S}) \tag{3}$$

where n is a binary random variable stating whether it is a herniated or a normal disc, S incorporates shape features extracted from both the GVF-snake and the ASM convergence. We utilize a Gibbs distribution with two shape potentials:

$$P(n|\mathsf{S}) = \frac{1}{Z[n]} \exp^{-[\alpha_1 U_{\mathsf{S}1} + \alpha_2 U_{\mathsf{S}2}]} \tag{4}$$

where S represents the shape features extracted from both the ASM convergence and the GVF-snake, $Z[n]$ is the normalization factor of the Gibbs distribution, α_1 and α_2 are tuning parameters. We define two shape potentials: (1) U_{S1} models the GVF-snake delineation for the posterior segment of the disc. (2) U_{S2} models the major axis of the ASM converged disc shape.

We extract the first shape potential U_{S1} from the GVF-snake delineation of the posterior disc segment. The longer the contour, the more likely it delineates a herniated segment as shown in Fig. 5 by the yellow line between the points k_1 and k_9. To capture the length of the GVF-snake contour, we model the number of points that are sampled by the final GVF-contour. The GVF-snake interpolates the pixels by having a maximum of two pixels between each point. Thus, we define:

$$U_{S1} = \frac{\left(e_1 - \mu_{e_1}\right)^2}{2\sigma_{e_1}^2} \tag{5}$$

where e_1 is the number of interpolated points along the delineated GVF contour, μ_{e_1} $\sigma_{e_1}^2$ are the expected and the variance of the interpolated points on the GVF-contour, respectively. We estimate both μ_{e_1} and $\sigma_{e_1}^2$ from the training data.

The secondary shape potential, U_{S2}, is motivated by the clinical observation that the herniated disc collapses due to the leak of the nucleus pulposus causing average lengthening in the major axis of the disc as shown in Fig. 1. We utilize this by incorporating this second shape potential U_{S2}:

$$U_{S2} = \frac{\left(e_2 - \mu_{e_2}\right)^2}{2\sigma_{e_2}^2} \tag{6}$$

where e_2 is the disc major axis length, μ_{e_2} is the expected major axis length of the disc, $\sigma_{e_2}^2$ is the variance of the major axis length of the disc. We learn both μ_{e_2} and $\sigma_{e_2}^2$ from the training data. We define e_2 by:

$$e_2 = \left| \frac{k_1 + k_9}{2} - k_5 \right|_2 \tag{7}$$

where k_1, k_5, and k_9 are the location coordinates of points 1, 5, and 9, respectively, as shown in Fig. 4. The distance e_2 roughly measures the major disc axis length subtracting the average location of the right end points k_1 and k_9 and the left end point k_5.

3 Data and Results

Our clinical MRI dataset is captured by a Philips 3-Tesla scanner according to the clinical standard. Each case contains manually co-registered two sagittal views (T1- and T2-weighted) as well as six axial T1-weighted slices for each disc. We use the

Table 1 Cross validation results: each row tests randomly selected 35 cases

Set	L5-S1	L4-5	L3-4	L2-3	L1-2	T12-L1	Accuracy (%)
1	32	32	34	34	35	34	95.7
2	33	32	32	31	34	35	93.8
3	33	34	32	33	33	34	94.8
4	31	30	32	33	33	34	91.9
5	31	32	32	33	34	33	92.9
6	33	32	32	31	32	33	91.9
7	33	32	34	34	33	33	94.8
8	30	31	32	31	34	33	91.0
9	30	33	34	34	35	35	95.7
10	32	33	34	34	34	35	96.2
(%)	90.9	91.7	93.7	93.7	96.3	96.9	–
Average Accuracy							**93.9**

clinical diagnosis reports to obtain our diagnosis gold standard. We validate our proposed method on 65 subjects with ages of 23–76 years old and with various types of abnormalities. We perform a cross-validation experiment where we leave 35 cases for testing and use the remaining 30 for training. We perform 10 rounds and each time, we randomly select the training and testing cases. We define the accuracy in each round (row in the Table 1) as the sum of correctly classified discs $Accuracy_i = (1 - \frac{1}{M}\sum_{j=1}^{K}|g_{ij} - n_{ij}|) \times 100\%$ where i is the lumbar disc level, $1 \leq i \leq 6$, M is the testing set size in each round (35 cases).

Table 1 shows the classification results from the cross validation experiment. We achieve an average of 93.9% accuracy on disc diagnosis. Each row in the table represents one round of the cross-validation. Thus, it represents 35 cases with 6 discs each case. We show the number of correctly classified discs at each disc level (column) out of 35 discs. We further compute the overall specificity and sensitivity where:

$$Specificity = \frac{TN}{TN + FP} \tag{8}$$

$$Sensitivity = \frac{TP}{TP + FN} \tag{9}$$

where FP is the number of false positives (normal discs diagnosed as herniated), TP is the number of true positives (correctly diagnosed herniated discs), FN is the number of false negatives (misclassified herniated discs), and TN is the number of true negatives (correctly classified normal discs). Table 2 shows another cross validation experiment with 15 randomly selected cases for 10 rounds. This makes 15×6 (discs) $\times 10$ (rounds) $= 900$ discs total (including repetitions). Within this cross validation experiment, there is a total of 78 misclassified discs: 25 herniated (false negatives) and 53 normal (false positives) as shown in Table 2. We archive an overall specificity over 92% and sensitivity over 87%.

Table 2 Calculation of specificity (96.6 %) and sensitivity (86.4 %)

		Gold standard Herniated	Normal
Result	Herniated	170 (TP)	53 (FP)
	Normal	25 (FN)	652 (TN)

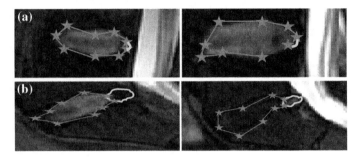

Fig. 6 Resulting ASM convergence and GVF-snake delineation for two normal cases and two abnormal ones

Figure 6 shows four examples from our dataset. It shows the convergence of the ASM point distribution (red dots and the linear connections) as well as the GVF-snake delineation (yellow curve). On the other hand, we compare our classification results to a Bayesian classifier that only models the disc appearance to show the effectiveness of modeling the shape. We run the same experiment with the same cases of Table 2 and obtain around 80 % average classification accuracy. We justify that by the fact that despite Herniated discs produce lower intensity levels; in general, the difference in intensity with the normal disc is not enough to classify herniated and normal discs. However, a Bayesian intensity-based classifier can be useful for other diseases such as disc desiccation [20]. Figure 6c shows a sample Herniated disc, with high intensity value, that was misclassified by the intensity-based classifier but correctly classified with our shape-based classifier.

4 Conclusion

We proposed a method for herniation diagnosis from lumbar area clinical MRI. We utilize a coordinated active shape and a gradient vector flow active contour models to extract shape features for detection of herniation. We use a Bayesian classifier and utilize a Gibbs-based distribution with shape potentials. We validate our method on a set of sixty five clinical MRI cases. We achieve an average of 93.9 % classification accuracy with specificity 96.6 % and sensitivity of 86.4 %. We also compared our results with the two state-of-the-art work and substantially outperform both of them due to our features that encompass the benefits of both works into a more robust classification model.

Acknowledgments This research was funded in part by NSF Grants DBI 0959870 and CNS 0855220 and NYSTAR grants 60701 and 41702.

References

1. Crow, W.T., Willis, D.R.: Estimating cost of care for patients with acute low back pain: a retrospective review of patient records. J. Am. Osteopath. Assoc. **109**(4), 229–233 (2009)
2. Nelson, J., O'Neil, C., Richardson, C.J.: Treatment of low back pain: exploring the costs. Health and Wellness (2012)
3. NINDS: National institute of neurological disorders and stroke (ninds): Low back pain fact sheet. NIND brochure (2008)
4. van Rijn, J.C., Klemets, N., Reitsma, J.B., Majoie, C.B.L.M., Hulsmans, F.J., Peul, W.C., Stam, J., Bossuyt, P.M., den Heeten, G.J.: Observer variation in MRI evaluation of patients suspected of lumbar disk herniation. AJR Am. J. Roentgenol. **184**(1), 299–303 (2005)
5. Atlas, S.J., Deyo, R.A.: Evaluating and managing acute low back pain in the primary care setting. J. Gen. Intern. Med. **16**(2), 120–131 (2011)
6. Swarm: Interactive incorporation (viewmedica)—patient educatuion system. (2007)
7. Fardon, D.F., Milette, P.C.: Nomenclature and classification of lumbar disc pathology. SPINE **26**(5), E93–E113 (2001)
8. Snell, R.S.: Clinical Anatomy by Regions. 8th edn. Lippincott, Williams & Wilkins, Philadelphia, Baltimore (2007)
9. Alomari, R.S., Corso, J.J., Chaudhary, V., Dhillon, G.: Toward a clinical lumbar CAD: herniation diagnosis. Int. J. Comput. Assist. Radiol. Surg. **6**, 119–126 (2011)
10. Alomari, R.S., Corso, J.J., Chaudhary, V., Dhillon, G.: Automatic diagnosis of lumbar disc herniation with shape and appearance features from MRI. In: Proceedings of SPIE Conference on Medical Imaging (SPIE) (2010)
11. Michopoulou, S., Costaridou, L., Panagiotopoulos, E., Speller, R., Panayiotakis, G., Todd-Pokropek, A.: Atlas-based segmentation of degenerated lumbar intervertebral discs from mr images of the spine. IEEE Trans. Biomed. Imaging **56**(9), 2225–2231 (2009)
12. Bounds, D., Lloyd, P., Mathew, B., Waddell, G.: A multilayer perceptron network for the diagnosis of low back pain. In: Proceedings of IEEE International Conference on Neural Networks, vol. 2, pp 481–489. San Diego, (1988)
13. Vaughn, M.: Using an artificial neural network to assist orthopaedic surgeons in the diagnosis of low back pain. http://www.marilyn-vaughn.co.uk/lbpainresearchstudy.htm (2000)
14. Tsai, M.D., Jou, S.B., Hsieh, M.S.: A new method for lumbar herniated inter-vertebral disc diagnosis based on image analysis of transverse sections. Comput. Med. Imaging Graph. **26**(6), 369–380 (2002)
15. Alomari, R.S., Corso, J.J., Chaudhary, V.: Labeling of lumbar discs using both pixel- and object-level features with a two-level probabilistic model. IEEE Trans. Med. Imaging **30**(1), 1–10 (2011)
16. Corso, J.J., Alomari, R.S., Chaudhary, V.: Lumbar disc localization and labeling with a probabilistic model on both pixel and object features. In: Proceedings of Medical Image Computing and Computer Aided Intervention (MICCAI). LNCS Part 1. vol 5241, pp. 202–210. Springer, Berlin (2008)
17. Cootes, T.F., Taylor, C.J.: Statistical models of appearance for medical image analysis and computer vision. In: Proceedings of SPIE Conference on Medical, Imaging (SPIE). pp. 236–248 (2001)

18. Xu, C., Prince, J.L.: Handbook of Medical Imaging. Academic, Baltimore (2000)
19. Liu, F., Zhao, B., Kijewski, P., Wang, L., Schwartz, L.: Liver segmentation for CT images using GVF snake. Med. Phys. **32**(12), 3699–3706 (2005)
20. Alomari, R.S., Corso, J.J., Chaudhary, V., Dhillon, G.: Desiccation diagnosis in lumbar discs from clinical MRI with a probabilistic model. In: Proceedings of IEEE International Symposium on Biomedical, Imaging (ISBI). pp. 546–549 (2009)

Epidural Masses Detection on Computed Tomography Using Spatially-Constrained Gaussian Mixture Models

Sanket Pattanaik, Jiamin Liu, Jianhua Yao, Weidong Zhang, Evrim Turkbey, Xiao Zhang and Ronald Summers

Abstract The widespread use of CT imaging and the critical importance of early detection of epidural masses of the spinal canal generate a scenario ideal for the implementation of a computer-aided detection (CAD) system. Epidural masses can lead to paralysis, incontinence and loss of neurological function if not promptly detected. We present, to our knowledge, the first CAD system to detect epidural masses on CT. In this paper, global intensity and local spatial features are modeled as spatially constrained Gaussian Mixture Model (CGMM) for epidural mass detection. The Cross-validation on 23 patients with epidural masses on body CT showed that the CGMM yielded a marked improvement of performance (69 % at 8.6 false positives per patient) over an intensity based K-means method (46 % at 7.9 false-positives per patient).

S. Pattanaik · J. Liu (✉) · J. Yao · W. Zhang · E. Turkbey · X. Zhang · R. Summers
Radiology and Imaging Sciences Department, Clinical Center,
The National Institutes of Health, Bethesda, MD 20892, USA
e-mail: liujiamin@cc.nih.gov

S. Pattanaik
e-mail: Sanket.Pattanaik@gmail.com

J. Yao
e-mail: jyao@cc.nih.gov

W. Zhang
e-mail: wdongzhang@gmail.com

E. Turkbey
e-mail: turkbeye@cc.nih.gov

X. Zhang
e-mail: zhangxn@cc.nih.gov

R. Summers
e-mail: rsummers@cc.nih.gov

J. Yao et al. (eds.), *Computational Methods and Clinical Applications
for Spine Imaging*, Lecture Notes in Computational Vision and Biomechanics 17,
DOI: 10.1007/978-3-319-07269-2_9, © Springer International Publishing Switzerland 2014

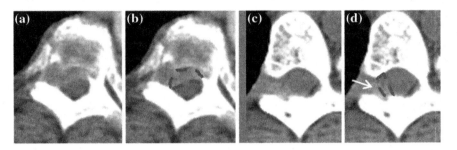

Fig. 1 Masses encroaching on epidural space of the spinal canal. Mass results in spinal stenosis and, atleast in (**a**, **b**), spinal cord compression. Epidural components of the masses are demarcated with *yellow dots*. **a**, **b** Osteolytic lesions can extend into epidural space. **c**, **d** Neural foramina, indicated by an *arrow*, can serve as another avenue for canal invasion

1 Introduction

Masses in the epidural space of the spinal canal can cause discomfort, pain and even paralysis by compressing the spinal cord and nerve roots. Moreover, the presence of an epidural mass within the spinal canal is a strong predictor of metastatic disease. A retrospective study of 337 patients at the Mayo Clinic, for instance, revealed that 20 % of all cases of spinal epidural metastases presented as the initial manifestations of malignancy [1]. Given the importance that early indicators of malignant cancers hold in the radiology community, the absence of a body of work on computer aided detection (CAD) of spinal canal lesions within the intradural and extradural space is quite surprising.

A CAD system designed to detect epidural masses within the constraints of the CT modality could prove invaluable. While confirmation of epidural tumors is almost always made using magnetic resonance imaging (MRI), due to its higher anatomic resolution and sensitivity to alterations of the central nervous system tissue, most patients will have received an examination using CT images. CT imaging remains the most prevalent radiologic modality as it is rapid (current generation can take less than 1 min), cost-effective, and can image over a large body area, effectively localizing many types of soft tissue tumors [2]. Automated detection of an epidural mass is very challenging because of its low contrast to normal soft tissue in the spinal canal. Even a radiologist may fail to detect an epidural mass in CT scan, especially when the patient is being examined for unrelated complications. Figure 1 shows examples of masses that are far more subtle in the CT scan and detectable as a slightly hyper-attenuating region when the image is viewed using an appropriate soft-tissue window width and level. In fact, the patient cohort examined in this study had an MRI confirming the presence of an epidural mass nearly a month after the mass was detectable on a CT scan, a duration that could drastically affect patient outcome when concerning progressive disease.

A vast majority of tumors that encroach on the epidural spaces originate from the intravertebral foramina or the vertebral bodies surrounding the spinal canal [3].

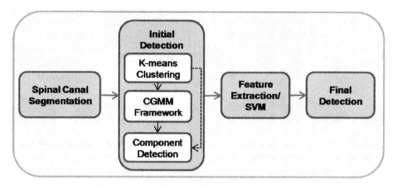

Fig. 2 Workflow

In other words, the masses always extend contiguously from the radiopaque bony regions of the spine into the soft tissue and can be discriminated as an intermediate tissue existing between bone and soft tissue. In this work, these spatial constraints are incorporated into conventional intensity based Gaussian mixture model (GMM) as a spatially-constrained Gaussian mixture model (CGMM) [4] for epidural mass detection. A large number of Gaussians is used per tissue in the spinal canal to capture the local spatial feature. The intensity of a tissue is considered a global feature and is modeled by parameters linking all associated Gaussians.

2 Methods

Our method involves the segmentation of the spinal canal and vertebral components of the spine, expansion and refinement of the spinal canal, a mass candidate detection phase, and feature computation and selection phase for support vector machine (SVM) classification. Within the detection phase of the protocol, intensity based K-means clustering is used for initial classification of tissues in the spinal canal, including the epidural masses. Then a CGMM framework is implemented to refine the tissue classification for accurate mass detection. Figure 2 shows the workflow of our procedure.

2.1 Region of Interest Detection

Segmentation of the spinal canal proceeded first with whole spine segmentation, using the watershed algorithm followed by a directed graph search [5]. A four-part vertebra model was then used to locate the vertebral bodies, spinous processes, and left/right transverse processes, with rib structures used to separate vertebral segments.

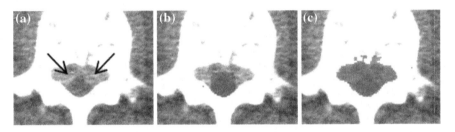

Fig. 3 Epidural mass (**a**) is not included in initial segmentation of the spinal canal (**b**), but is included in modified canal segmentation (**c**)

Curved planar reformations were then employed to segment the spinal canal, using the centerline as a backbone [5]. One example of segmented spinal canal is shown in Fig. 3b.

The segmentation of the spinal canal, however, suffers from the ambiguity in discriminating between hyper-attenuating bony and spinal lesion regions within the canal. As a result, many cases under-segment the region of interest within which we expect to detect epidural masses. To contend with this complication, we modified the initial segmentation of the spinal canal by dilating (by 7 mm), thresholding (by 250 HU), and performing connect component analysis to extend the segmentation so that it encompasses the epidural masses. The expansion is demonstrated in Fig. 3c. Expansion of the canal ensured hyperintense masses were included within our search region as were the intravertebral foraminae, which often serves as a source point for epidural masses [3].

2.2 K-Means Clustering for Initial Classification

Classification by clustering the intensities of the voxels within the region of interest into $k = 5$ different classes, or K-Means clustering, makes full use of our prior understanding of the arrangements of constituent tissues of the spinal canal. Selecting four different classes allowed us to delineate classes representative of normal intradural soft tissue, hypo-attenuating fatty tissue and vasculature [3], epidural masses, and the partial volume between the bone and soft tissue. An additional fifth class was included to contain bony voxels that had not been successfully removed.

2.3 CGMM for Tissue Classification Refinement

The CGMM framework was modified from a method [4] employed to detect multiple sclerosis lesions from MRI images of the brain. To accommodate the spatial feature, we model an image as if its voxels were drawn independently from a mixture of many Gaussians:

$$f(x, I(x)) = \sum_{i=1}^{n} \alpha_i f_i(x, I(x)|\mu_i, \Sigma_i) \tag{1}$$

where x is the 3D position information included in the spatial vector (spatial parameters), $I(x)$ is the intensity vector (intensity parameters) associated with the voxel in position x, n is the number of Gaussians components in the mixture model, μ_i and Σ_i are the mean and the covariance of the ith Gaussian components f_i, and α_i is the ith mixture coefficient. The spatial feature is incorporated into the probabilistic model. Each Gaussian component in the CGMM represents a probabilistic model for a specific small area in the CT image, therefore $n \gg k$. Each Gaussian component is linked to a single tissue class and all the Gaussian components related to the same tissue class share the same intensity parameters. Assuming the intensity and spatial features are uncorrelated, we have

$$\mu_i = \begin{pmatrix} \mu_i^x \\ \mu_{\pi(i)}^I \end{pmatrix}, \ \Sigma_i = \begin{pmatrix} \Sigma_i^x & 0 \\ 0 & \Sigma_{\pi(i)}^I \end{pmatrix} \tag{2}$$

$\pi(i)$ is the tissue that is linked to the ith Gaussian component, μ_i^x and Σ_i^x are the spatial mean and covariance of the ith Gaussian component, and $\mu_{\pi(i)}^I$ and $\Sigma_{\pi(i)}^I$ are intensity mean and variance of class $\pi(1 \leq \pi \leq 5)$ to which the ith Gaussian component belongs. Therefore, the Gaussian component f_i can be writte as:

$$f(x, I(x)) = \sum_{i=1}^{n} \alpha_i \mathcal{N}(x; \mu_i^x, \Sigma_i^x) \times \mathcal{N}(I(x); \mu_{\pi(i)}^I, \Sigma_{\pi(i)}^I) \tag{3}$$

The main advantage of the CGMM is to combine local spatial features with a global intensity feature, which makes the CGMM much more robust to noise than intensity based methods. The five tissue classes generated from the K-Means clustering served as the initialization for our CGMM framework. Small clusters(<20 voxels) were defined as under-representative of the associated tissue class. From the remaining clusters, 1/20 voxels were selected as center of Gaussian components in Eq. (1). Each voxel within the cluster was then linked to its nearest Gaussian center. The component coefficient α_i was then initialized as the number of voxels in ith Gaussian component divided by the total number of voxels of all n Gaussian components.

The spatial and intensity parameters were then recalculated using the Expectation-Maximization (EM) algorithm. As explicated by Freifeld et al. [4], the parameters are retrieved by iterating through an expectation step followed by a maximization step. Within the expectation step, an initial prediction of the parameters (starting with the initialization provided from the five tissue classes generated by the K-means clustering) is made. The posterior probability of a voxel t [4], originating from the ith Gaussian component, is given by

$$p(i|x_t, I(x_t)) = \frac{\alpha_i f_i(x, I(x)|\mu_i, \Sigma_i)}{\sum_{j=1}^{n} \alpha_i f_j(x, I(x)|\mu_j, \Sigma_j)} \qquad i = 1:n, t = 1(\text{number of voxels})$$

(4)

The posterior probability is then used to re-estimate the means, covariance matrices, and component coefficients in the maximization step:

$$n_i = \sum_{t=1}^{T} p(i|x_t, I(x_t)) \quad i = 1:n,$$

(5)

$$k_j = \sum_{i|\pi(i)=j} n_i \quad j = 1:5$$

$$\alpha_i = n_i / (\text{total number of voxels})$$

where n_i and k_j represent the expected number of voxels associated with the ith mixture component and the kth tissue $(1 \le k \le 5)$.

Means:

$$\mu_i^x = \frac{1}{n_i} \sum_{t=1}^{T} p(i|x_t, I(x_t))x_t,$$

(6)

$$\mu_j^I = \frac{1}{k_j} \sum_{i|\pi(i)=j} \sum_{t=1}^{T} p(i|x_t, I(x_t))I(x_t)$$

Covariance Matrices:

$$\Sigma_i^x = \frac{1}{n_i} \sum_{t=1}^{T} p(i|x_t, I(x_t))(x_t - \mu_i^x)(x_t - \mu_i^x)^T,$$

(7)

$$\Sigma_j^I = \frac{1}{k_j} \sum_{i|\pi(i)=j} \sum_{t=1}^{T} p(i|x_t, I(x_t))(I(x_t) - \mu_j^I)(I(x_t) - \mu_j^I)^T$$

After applying EM for estimation of the spatial and intensity parameters of each Gaussian, a Maximum-A-Posteriori (MAP) criterion was used to return label L for each voxel t [4]:

$$L_t = arg \max_{j} \sum_{i|\pi(i)=j} \alpha_i f_i(x, I(x)|\mu_i, \Sigma_i)$$

(8)

As a result, five new tissue classes are generated. Figure 4 shows the classification by K-mean and CGMM. The detected epidural masses are used for feature computation and false positive reduction.

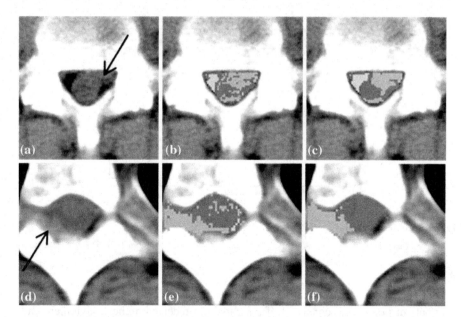

Fig. 4 Example of 5-tissue classification. **a, d** Epidural masses were confirmed on MRI and demarcated in CT images by radiologists. **b, e** K-Means clustering result (note 3 classes visible on images: soft tissue in *brown*; fat in *yellow*; epidural mass in *blue*). **c, f** CGMM-refined tissue classes, emphasizing large spatially confined components such as epidural masses

2.4 Feature Extraction and SVM

A comprehensive collection of texture features from the mass detections were computed in this work. Haralick Gray-Level Co-occurrence Matrix (GLCM) features [6] are widely used for analyzing image texture. The co-occurrence matrix stores the co-occurrence frequencies of the pairs of gray levels, which are configured by different distances and directions. We calculated the co-occurrence matrices for 4 offset distances and 13 directions on multiple planes, yielding 52 matrices for each mass detection. We then calculated 12 features from the matrix, including energy, entropy, correlation, contrast, variance, sum of mean, inertia, cluster shade, cluster tendency, homogeneity, maximal probability, and inverse variance. Thus, each detected mass has 624 Haralick GLCM features. We also extracted the volume of the masses, histograms of oriented gradients and local binary patterns features. Finally, an SVM committee [7] is employed to reduce false-positive detections. The method involved bootstrap aggregation of features into several SVM committees to improve on selection of features and avoid overfitting.

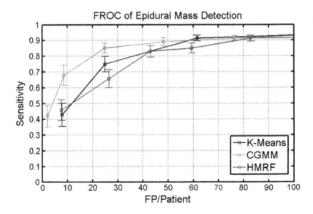

Fig. 5 10-fold cross validation FROC of three methods

3 Results

The patient population consisted of patients who received a chest, abdomen, and pelvis CT scan within 1 month before or after receiving an MRI confirming the presence of an epidural mass. A cohort of 23 patients, with a total of 54 epidural masses confirmed as visible in the CT images by radiologists, were examined in this study. The inter-slice spacing was 5 mm, and the voxel spacing within an axial slice was in the range 0.7–0.9 mm.The detected epidural mass was marked as true-positive if constituent voxels were within 10 mm of the epidural mass centroids demarcated as ground truth by a radiologist.

The detection performance was evaluated using ten-fold cross-validation. The free response receiver operating characteristic (FROC) curves of the detection performance are shown in Fig. 5. For example, we get a sensitivity of 46 % with 7.9 false positive per patient on average for K-means method. We achieve a sensitivity of 69 % with 8.6 false positives per patient on average for the CGMM method. The difference in the methods was statistically significant ($p = 0.02$) at the aforementioned operating points as determined using Fischer's exact test [8]. By contrast,the results from an existing Hidden Markov Random Fields (HMRF) method [9], which also incorporates spatial context information, is similar to the K-means method. Figure 6 shows examples of true and false positive, false negative detections. Of the three masses that were missed in our study, two of them appeared near the sacrum, where the spinal canal segmentation was arrested. The other was a large lytic lesion that spanned much of the intervertebral surface and extended to the mediastinum, disrupting the spine segmentation. A large number of false positive cases were located around the dorsal surface of the spinal canal, in a hyperattenuating channel within the vertebral body. This region contains the basivertebral vein [10], contributing to erroneous detection in the CAD.

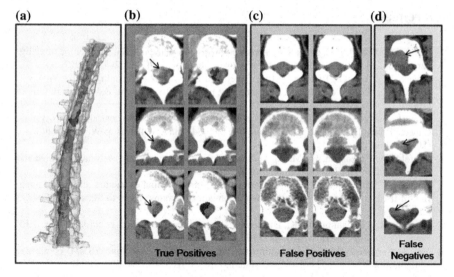

(a) (b) (c) (d)

True Positives   False Positives   False Negatives

Fig. 6 Examples of detections. **a** Result from CGMM of one patient (TP in *blue*; FP in *red*). Axial slices of **b** TP, **c** FP, and **d** FN (*arrow*) from several patients

4 Discussion

Our study reveals that K-Means clustering coupled with refinement CGMM is a viable preliminary approach to the detection of epidural masses in the CT imaging modality. This work illustrates the importance of considering spatial context in specific CAD problems, especially when the context can be mapped onto anatomically distinct tissues. We plan to explore how performance improves when using a much more informed prior for the spatial distribution of tissues. The epidural masses considered in this study all extend from the boundary of the spinal canal, a fact that could be used to improve the segmentation. Once segmentation of the masses is refined shape context information (such as sphericity) may be extracted to improve the performance of CAD. This could require implementation of curve-fitting algorithms attuned to the unique challenges posed by the difficulty of distinguishing epidural masses from soft tissue or bone. Lastly, stratification of CAD performance as it correlates with type of mass (if confirmed by biopsy) or degree of invasion or stenosis induced by the mass could lend unique insight into necessary modifications for a generalization of the system.

References

1. Schiff, D., O'Neill, B.P., et al.: Spinal epidural metastasis as the initial manifestation of malignancy: clinical features and diagnostic approach. Neurology **49**(2), 452–456 (1997)
2. Hricak, H., Akin, O., Bradbury, M.S.: Functional and metabolic imaging. In: DeVita, V.T. (ed.) Cancer: Principles & Practice of Oncology, pp. 589–616. Williams & Wilkins, Baltimore (2005)
3. Fine, H., Barker, F.G., Markert, J.M., Loeffler, J.S.: Neoplasms of the central nervous system. Cancer: Principles & Practice of Oncology, pp. 1834–1887. Williams & Wilkins, Baltimore (2005)
4. Freifeld, O., Greenspan, H.: Multiple sclerosis lesion detection using constrained GMM and curve evolution. Int. J. Biomed. Imaging **2009**, 14 (2009)
5. Jianhua, Y., O'Connor, S. D., et al.: Automated spinal column extraction and partitioning. In: 3rd IEEE International Symposium on Biomedical Imaging: Nano to Macro, pp 390–393 (2006)
6. Haralick, R.M., Shanmugam, K., Dinstein, I.: Textural features for image classification. IEEE Trans. Syst. Man Cybern. **3**, 610–621 (1973)
7. Yao, J., Summers, R.M., et al.: Optimizing the support vector machines (SVM) committee configuration in a colonic polyp CAD system. Proc. SPIE **5746**, 384–392 (2005)
8. Carlson, J., Heckerman, D., Shani, G.: False discovery rate for 2x2 contingency tables. Microsoft Research technical report MSR-TR-2009-53 (2009)
9. Wang, Q.: HMRF-EM-image: implementation of the Hidden Markov random field model and its expectation-maximization algorithm. CoRR e-prints (1207.3510)
10. Dorwart, R.H., DeGroot, J., Sauerland, E.T., et al.: CT of the lumbar spine: normal variants and pitfalls. Radiographics **2**(4), 459–499 (1982)

Part III
Quantitative Imaging

Comparison of Manual and Computerized Measurements of Sagittal Vertebral Inclination in MR Images

Tomaž Vrtovec, Franjo Pernuš and Boštjan Likar

Abstract In this study, sagittal vertebral inclination (SVI) was systematically measured by three observers for 28 vertebrae (T4-L5) from one normal and one scoliotic magnetic resonance (MR) spine image using six manual and two computerized measurements. Manual measurements were performed by superior and inferior tangents, anterior and posterior tangents, and mid-endplate and mid-wall lines. Computerized measurements were performed by automatically evaluating the symmetry of vertebral anatomy in sagittal cross-sections and volumetric images. The mid-wall lines were the manual measurements with the lowest intra- and inter-observer variability (1.4° and 1.9° standard deviation, SD). The strongest inter-method agreement was found between the mid-wall lines and posterior tangents (2.0° SD). Computerized measurements did not yield intra- and inter-observer variability (2.8° and 3.8° SD) as low as the mid-wall lines, but were still comparable to the intra- and inter-observer variability of the superior (2.6° and 3.7° SD) and inferior (3.2° and 4.5° SD) tangents.

1 Introduction

Spinal deformities are manifested in an altered orientation of vertebrae that can occur in sagittal, coronal and/or axial plane. Sagittal vertebral inclination (SVI) is the rotation of a vertebra projected onto the sagittal plane and is represented by kyphotic and lordotic spinal curvatures. A number of methods were proposed for its measurement in the form of sagittal spinal curvature, i.e. along multiple vertebrae [1–4], however,

T. Vrtovec (✉) · F. Pernuš · B. Likar
Faculty of Electrical Engineering, University of Ljubljana, Tržaška cesta 25,
SI-1000 Ljubljana, Slovenia
e-mail: tomaz.vrtovec@fe.uni-lj.si

F. Pernuš
e-mail: franjo.pernus@fe.uni-lj.si

B. Likar
e-mail: bostjan.likar@fe.uni-lj.si

J. Yao et al. (eds.), *Computational Methods and Clinical Applications
for Spine Imaging*, Lecture Notes in Computational Vision and Biomechanics 17,
DOI: 10.1007/978-3-319-07269-2_10, © Springer International Publishing Switzerland 2014

not all of them can be used to measure the sagittal inclination in the form of segmental vertebral angulation, i.e. for a single vertebra [5–8]. The inclination of superior and inferior vertebral endplates was proposed by Cobb [5] to measure the severity of scoliosis in coronal radiographs, and later adapted to measure SVI in sagittal radiographs. However, the "modified" Cobb angle measurements are strongly affected by endplate architecture [9], vertebral body shape [10] and deformities in the coronal plane [11]. Alternatively, measuring the inclination of vertebral body walls resulted in posterior [7] and anterior [8] tangents. A number of systematic analyses were performed to define reference SVI in normal spines [8, 12–14]. Stagnara et al. [12] concluded that "normal" sagittal curves do not exist, as the range of SVI in normal subjects was considerably large. Bernhardt and Bridwell [13] proposed to use ranges of inclination instead of mean values. Korovessis et al. [14] showed that thoracic kyphosis increases with age, whereas lumbar lordosis starts to decrease after the seventh decade of life. Schuler et al. [8] compared manual and computer-assisted measurements of SVI using seven different measurements on 10 radiographs of L4/L5 and L5/S1 segments. The manual and computer-assisted measurements proved to be equivalent in terms of variability, the Cobb angle and posterior tangents were the least variable, and the anterior tangents were the most reliable measurements. Street et al. [15] evaluated the reliability of measuring kyphosis manually from different imaging modalities in the case of thoracolumbar fractures. For the Cobb angle measurements, they concluded that plain radiographs were the most reliable measurement modality, followed by computed tomography (CT) and finally by magnetic resonance (MR) imaging.

In the above mentioned studies, the measurements were performed in two-dimensional (2D) sagittal radiographs. Over the past years, MR has gained acceptance in spine imaging by providing high-quality three-dimensional (3D) images by a correct selection of imaging parameters. When compared to plain radiography or CT, MR is associated with higher costs and not suitable for imaging subjects with metal implants as they cause distortions in the acquired images, however, it does not deliver ionizing radiation to the patients. When MR is available or required, additional imaging can be therefore avoided to contain costs and limit exposure to unnecessary ionizing radiation. As a result, MR images of the spine were already used to measure various vertebral parameters [15–22]. A number of methods were proposed to measure SVI in lateral radiographic projections, but the variability of SVI measurements in MR images has not been investigated yet. The purpose of this study is therefore to systematically analyze the variability of manual and computerized measurements of SVI in MR images.

2 Methodology

2.1 Manual Measurements

The following six manual measurements were used to evaluate SVI (Fig. 1). The *superior* and *inferior tangents* represent the Cobb method [5] at the superior and

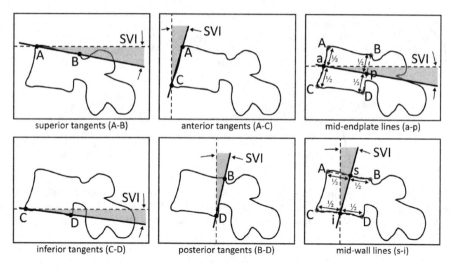

Fig. 1 The corners of the vertebral body (points *A*, *B*, *C* and *D*) in the sagittal view define the manual measurements of sagittal vertebral inclination (SVI)

inferior vertebral endplate, respectively. The *anterior* [8] and *posterior tangents* [7] represent the inclination of the anterior and posterior vertebral body wall, respectively. The *mid-endplate* and *mid-wall lines* are defined between the central points of the anterior and posterior vertebral body walls, and between the central points of the superior and inferior vertebral endplates, respectively. Each MR image was visualized by a specially developed computer program that allowed the observer to manually identify the vertebral centroid in 3D, and the coronal and axial vertebral rotation to extract a 2D oblique sagittal cross-section from the 3D image. In the oblique sagittal cross-section, the observer then manually identified the corners of each vertebral body that were used to determine the angles ω_x of SVI, measured against reference horizontal or vertical lines that are parallel to the coordinate system of the 3D image.

2.2 Computerized Measurements

Computerized measurements of SVI were performed by a method that determines vertebral rotation in 3D [23]. The rotation of a vertebra in a 3D image can be represented by the angles $\boldsymbol{\omega} = (\omega_x, \omega_y, \omega_z)$ of rotation of the local vertebral coordinate system V (defined by Cartesian unit vectors $\mathbf{e}_{V_x}$, $\mathbf{e}_{V_y}$ and $\mathbf{e}_{V_z}$) around the axes of the global image coordinate system I (defined by Cartesian unit vectors $\mathbf{e}_{I_x}$, $\mathbf{e}_{I_y}$ and $\mathbf{e}_{I_z}$). Both V and I are right-hand Cartesian coordinate systems, representing left-to-right (x-axis), anterior-to-posterior (y-axis) and cranial-to-caudal (z-axis) direction. The angles ω_x (i.e. SVI), ω_y (i.e. coronal vertebral inclination) and ω_z (i.e. axial vertebral rotation) then represent the rotation of the vertebral coordinate system V

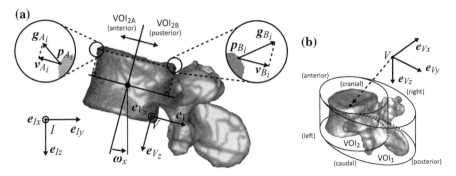

Fig. 2 **a** Example of symmetrical anatomical correspondence in anterior/posterior direction (S_y), shown for a symmetrical pair of points $\mathbf{p}_{A_i}$ and $\mathbf{p}_{B_i}$ inside VOI$_2$. **b** The vertebral coordinate system V and the observed volumes of interest (VOI$_1$ encompasses the whole vertebra, VOI$_2$ encompasses the vertebral body)

around vectors $\mathbf{e}_{I_x}$ (pitch), $\mathbf{e}_{I_y}$ (roll) and $\mathbf{e}_{I_z}$ (yaw), respectively. If the origin of V is located at the vertebral centroid and V is rotationally aligned with the vertebra in I, anatomically corresponding symmetrical parts of the vertebra can be observed within volumes of interest (VOIs) along positive/negative directions of each axis $\mathbf{e}_{V_j}$, $j = x, y, z$. The angles $\boldsymbol{\omega}$ of vertebral rotation can be therefore determined by finding the planes of maximal symmetry, which divide the whole vertebra into symmetrical left/right ($\pm\mathbf{e}_{V_x}$) halves, and the vertebral body into symmetrical anterior/posterior ($\pm\mathbf{e}_{V_y}$) and cranial/caudal ($\pm\mathbf{e}_{V_z}$) halves. For each axis $\mathbf{e}_{V_j}$, $j = x, y, z$, the symmetrical correspondences of the two halves (A and B) of a VOI are measured by $S_j(\text{VOI})$:

$$S_j(\text{VOI}) = \frac{\sum_{i=1}^{N} |\mathbf{v}_{A_i}| \cdot |\mathbf{v}_{B_i}| \cdot f}{\sum_{i=1}^{N} |\mathbf{v}_{A_i}| \cdot \sum_{i=1}^{N} |\mathbf{v}_{B_i}|}; \qquad f = \begin{cases} 1; & \mathbf{v}_{A_i} \cdot \mathbf{v}_{B_i} < 0 \\ 0; & \text{otherwise}, \end{cases} \tag{1}$$

where f is the weighting function, and $\mathbf{v}_{A_i}$ and $\mathbf{v}_{B_i}$ are the projections of the intensity gradient vectors $\mathbf{g}_{A_i}$ and $\mathbf{g}_{B_i}$ in the coordinate system I to the unit vector $\mathbf{e}_{V_j}$, $j = x, y, z$, of the coordinate system V at symmetrical pair of points $\mathbf{p}_{A_i}$ and $\mathbf{p}_{B_i}$, respectively, and N is the number of point pairs inside each VOI (Fig. 2a). By projecting the gradient vectors to $\mathbf{e}_{V_j}$, $j = x, y, z$, and by applying the weighting function f, we retain the gradient components $\mathbf{v}_{A_i}$ and $\mathbf{v}_{B_i}$ that are relevant for defining the vertebral symmetry in the direction of $\mathbf{e}_{V_j}$. Two variations of the computerized method were applied for each vertebra. The *measurements in 3D* automatically evaluated the vertebral rotation in 3D images by maximizing symmetrical correspondences:

$$\omega_x^* = \arg_{\omega_x}(\boldsymbol{\omega}); \quad \omega^* = \arg\max_{\omega}\left(S_x(\text{VOI}_1) + S_y(\text{VOI}_2) + S_z(\text{VOI}_2)\right), \tag{2}$$

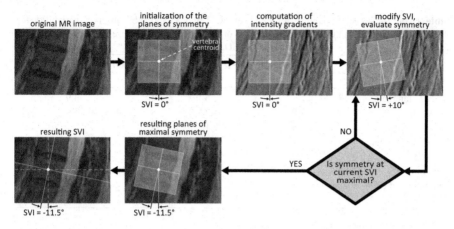

original MR image | initialization of the planes of symmetry | computation of intensity gradients | modify SVI, evaluate symmetry

vertebral centroid

SVI = 0° | SVI = 0° | SVI = +10°

resulting SVI | resulting planes of maximal symmetry | NO

YES | Is symmetry at current SVI maximal?

SVI = -11.5° | SVI = -11.5°

Fig. 3 An illustration of the computerized search for the coronal (anterior/posterior) and axial (cranial/caudal) planes of maximal symmetry, which define the sagittal vertebral inclination (SVI), in a 2D oblique sagittal MR cross-section of the L1 vertebra

where the VOI that encompasses the whole vertebra is denoted by VOI_1, and the VOI that encompasses the vertebral body is denoted by VOI_2 (Fig. 2b). On the other hand, the *measurements in 2D* automatically evaluated SVI in the same 2D oblique sagittal cross-sections that were used for manual measurements (Fig. 3) by considering only VOI_2 that encompasses the vertebral body and reducing its dimensionality to the area of interest (AOI), and maximizing the remaining symmetrical correspondences:

$$\omega_x^* = \arg\max_{\omega_x^*} \big(S_y(\mathrm{AOI}) + S_z(\mathrm{AOI})\big). \tag{3}$$

The planes of symmetry are first manually initialized so that they are parallel to the 3D axes of the MR image, centered in the vertebral centroid in 3D, and 50 mm in size to encompass the whole vertebral body of thoracic and lumbar segments. By rotating these planes in 3D, the rotation angles ω_x^* are obtained from the inclination of the planes, and the current symmetrical correspondences are evaluated by mirroring the edges of vertebral anatomical structures (obtained from image intensity gradients) over each plane and comparing them to the edges on the opposite side of that plane in an optimization procedure.

3 Experiments and Results

3.1 Images and Observers

A total of $n = 28$ vertebrae between segments T4 and L5 from one normal (28-year male, 1° frontal Cobb angle) and one scoliotic (25-year male, 14° frontal

Table 1 Intra-observer variability for observers 1, 2 and 3, and inter-observer variability for observer pairs 1-2, 1-3 and 2-3 when performing or initializing sagittal vertebral inclination (SVI) measurements, reported as standard deviations (SD, in degrees)

Method	Intra-observer SD				Inter-observer SD			
	1	2	3	Mean	1-2	1-3	2-3	Mean
Superior tangents	3.1	2.1	2.5	2.6	3.4	3.8	3.9	3.7
Inferior tangents	4.3	2.2	2.6	3.2	4.8	4.7	3.9	4.5
Anterior tangents	2.1	1.4	2.6	2.1	2.5	3.2	2.9	2.9
Posterior tangents	1.8	1.1	2.0	1.7	2.3	2.7	2.3	2.4
Mid-endplate lines	2.1	1.5	1.4	1.7	2.8	2.7	2.9	2.8
Mid-wall lines	1.3	1.0	1.8	1.4	1.7	2.1	2.0	1.9
Computerized (2D)	2.0	1.4	4.1	2.8	2.2	4.4	4.3	3.8
Computerized (3D)	3.4	4.1	1.1	3.1	5.8	5.5	4.2	5.2

Cobb angle) spine image were included in this study. The T2-weighted MR scans (mean repetition and echo time $TR = 4,560$ ms and $TE = 102$ ms, matrix size 512×512, field of view 200×200 mm^2, slice thickness 3 mm) were acquired by a spine array coil with a 1.5 T Signa Excite MR Scanner (GE Healthcare, Milwaukee, WI, USA). Three observers with different experience in medical imaging and orthopedic surgery (observer 1: a postgraduate biomedical engineering student, observer 2: a medical imaging researcher, observer 3: a spine surgeon) independently performed two series of measurements that were 2 weeks apart.

3.2 Results

The intra-observer variability in terms of standard deviation (SD) of observers 1, 2 and 3 was 2.6°, 1.6° and 2.2°, respectively, for manual measurements, and 2.8°, 3.1° and 3.0°, respectively, for computerized measurements (Table 1). The overall intra-observer variability was therefore estimated to 2.1° for manual and 3.0° for computerized measurements. There were no statistically significant differences between the first and second series of measurements for each observer ($p > 0.49$; independent-samples t-test with the level of significance $\alpha = 0.05$). The inter-observer variability in terms of SD of observer pairs 1-2, 1-3 and 2-3 was 3.1°, 3.3° and 3.1°, respectively, for manual measurements, and 4.4°, 5.0° and 4.3°, respectively, for computerized measurements (Table 1). The overall inter-observer variability was therefore estimated to 3.2° for manual and 4.6° for computerized measurements. There were no statistically significant differences between the measurements for each observer pair ($p > 0.63$; independent-samples t-test with the level of significance $\alpha = 0.05$). The comparison of SVI measurements is, in terms of agreement and difference between each pair of measurements, presented in Table 2, which also reports the obtained statistically significant differences between the measurement methods.

Table 2 Inter-method variability (lower-left in normal text) and difference (upper-right in bold text) of sagittal vertebral inclination (SVI) measurements, reported respectively as standard deviations (SD) and mean absolute differences (MAD) of the measured angles (in degrees)

	Superior tangents	Inferior tangents	Anterior tangents	Posterior tangents	Mid-end-plate lines	Mid-wall lines	Computer-ized (2D)	Computer-ized (3D)
Superior tangents	×	**3.5**	**3.2**†	**2.0**	**1.8**	**2.2**	**3.8**‡	**4.5**
Inferior tangents	5.9	×	**4.1**†	**4.1**	**1.7**	**3.9**†	**4.2**‡	**4.0**
Anterior tangents	3.4†	4.8†	×	**2.5**	**3.2**†	**1.3**	**2.9**	**3.5**
Posterior tangents	3.1	6.1	3.2	×	**2.8**	**1.3**	**2.8**†	**4.1**
Mid-endplate lines	3.5	3.7	2.9†	3.8	×	**2.7**†	**3.7**†	**3.7**
Mid-wall lines	2.9	5.2†	2.1	2.0	3.0†	×	**2.6**	**3.4**
Computer-ized (2D)	4.7‡	6.3‡	4.7	4.5†	4.7†	4.4	×	**3.9**
Computer-ized (3D)	6.3	7.3	6.0	5.9	6.1	5.8	5.8	×

† $p < 0.05$; ‡ $p < 0.001$

4 Discussion

4.1 Manual Measurements

For manual SVI measurements, the intra-observer variability was in general higher for observer 1 than for observers 2 and 3, while the inter-observer variability was in general lower for observer pair 1-2 than for observer pairs 1-3 and 2-3. Such results indicate that both clinical and imaging experience may be important for achieving reproducible measurements, while imaging experience may be important for achieving reliable measurements. The mid-wall lines proved to be the most reproducible and also the most reliable manual measurements (SD of 1.4° and 1.9°, respectively), followed by the posterior tangents (SD of 1.7° and 2.4°, respectively) and mid-endplate lines (SD of 1.7° and 2.8°, respectively). However, such results may be biased by the fact that the mid-wall and mid-endplate lines are determined by all identified points (i.e. the four corners of vertebral body). On the other hand, the relatively high reproducibility and reliability of the posterior tangents indicate that the posterior corners of the vertebral body may be identified more accurately than the anterior corners. The least repeatable and reliable manual measurements were the superior tangents (SD of 2.6° and 3.7°, respectively) and inferior tangents (SD of 3.2° and 4.5°, respectively). It was already shown that endplate architecture [9], vertebral body shape [10] and deformities in the coronal plane [11] can affect these measurements. In a recent evaluation of the same six manual measurements performed in CT images [24], it was reported that the mid-wall lines are also the most reproducible (1.0° SD) and reliable (1.4° SD), while the superior and inferior tangents are also the least reproducible (1.8° and 1.5° SD, respectively) and reliable (2.5° and 2.0° SD, respectively) manual measurements. These findings indicate that, although the variability was lower for CT images, the performance of a specific measurement is not considerably affected if measurements are obtained from MR or CT images.

4.2 Computerized Measurements

For computerized SVI measurements, the intra-observer and inter-observer variability of the measurements in 2D (SD of 2.8° and 3.8°, respectively) and of the measurements in 3D (SD of 3.1° and 5.2°, respectively) were in general as high as for the least repeatable and reliable manual measurements. Although computerized measurements in general provide more accurate and less variable results, the present study shows that such properties were not achieved when measuring SVI in MR images by the applied computerized method [23]. On the other hand, measurements in CT images [24] resulted in relatively low intra-observer and inter-observer variability (0.9° and 1.6° SD, respectively, for the measurements in 2D), which may be induced by the fact that the edges of bone structures can be extracted more accurately from CT than from MR images. Higher variability of the computerized measurements in 3D may originate from the fact that the measurements in 3D are more computationally demanding and error-prone than the measurements in 2D, as three rotation angles are simultaneously evaluated in 3D compared to the evaluation of only one rotation angle in 2D. However, the measurements in 2D had to be initialized in the manually identified vertebral centroids in 3D with known coronal and axial vertebral rotation, while the initialization of the measurements in 3D required only the vertebral centroids in 3D, which represents a considerable reduction in the effort of the observers.

4.3 Comparison of Measurements

Among manual measurements, the highest agreement was found between the mid-wall lines and posterior tangents (2.0° SD and 1.3° MAD), and between the mid-wall lines and anterior tangents (2.1° SD and 1.3° MAD). Such findings are not surprising, since the mid-wall lines represent a compromise between the anterior and posterior tangents, however, the agreement between the latter was lower (3.2° SD and 2.5° MAD). Although mid-endplate lines represent a compromise between the superior and inferior tangents, the agreement between the mid-endplate lines and superior tangents (3.5° SD and 1.8° MAD), between the mid-endplate lines and inferior tangents (3.7° SD and 1.7° MAD), and between the superior and inferior tangents (5.9° SD and

3.5°MAD) was considerably lower, which confirms that vertebral endplates represent unreliable anatomical references [9–11]. When comparing manual to computerized measurements, the strongest agreement was observed between the computerized measurements in 2D and mid-wall lines (4.4° SD and 2.6° MAD), and between the computerized measurements in 2D and posterior tangents (4.5° SD and 2.8° MAD). The agreement between manual measurements and the computerized measurements in 3D was in general lower. Similar findings were obtained in the study of SVI in CT images [24], where the computerized measurements were most consistent with lines parallel to vertebral body walls (i.e. anterior tangents, posterior tangents and mid-wall lines). However, manual and computerized measurements were based on completely different principles (i.e. the location of distinctive anatomical points vs. the symmetry of anatomical structures), and none can be assumed to represent the reference SVI.

4.4 Statistical Evaluation

The main limitation of the performed study is that the number of vertebrae for which SVI was evaluated is relatively low. Considering the obtained variabilities in the form of SD, the sample size $n = 28$ and the level of significance $\alpha = 0.05$ with the corresponding standard score $z_{\alpha/2} = 1.96$ that returns the probability $P(z > 1.96) = \alpha/2$, it can be assumed with 95 % confidence that the mean difference of the sample is within $\pm E$ of the mean difference of the population, where $E = SD \cdot z_{\alpha/2}/\sqrt{n}$. By considering that the difference of $E = \pm 1°$ is practically acceptable, the given sample size results in the SD of 2.7°. As is can be observed from Tables 1 and 2, the obtained SDs are sometimes below, but in general above 2.7°, meaning that a larger sample size would be required for the desired mean difference of the sample. However, the measurements were acquired as part of a larger study of vertebral rotation in 3D, where besides SVI, also coronal vertebral inclination and axial vertebral rotation were systematically evaluated in MR [21, 22] and CT [24, 25] images. As manual measurements were relatively time-consuming, the number of vertebrae was therefore limited so that the observers could perform each series of measurements at once, i.e. without breaks that could bias their measurement strategy or judgment. The current results may be therefore interpreted as a pilot study that is useful to obtain an estimation of the SD of the measurements. Therefore, if the SD for SVI measurement in MR images is around 5°, the adequate sample size is around 100, which can be regarded as a guideline for future work.

5 Conclusion

In conclusion, SVI was evaluated in MR images using six manual and two computerized measurements. The mid-wall lines, defined by four distinct anatomical points, proved to be the manual measurements with the lowest intra- and inter-observer variability. Posterior tangents yielded similar results and, as defined by only two points, they may represent an easier alternative for the observers. In addition, the lowest inter-method variability was found between the mid-wall lines and posterior tangents. Computerized measurements, based on the evaluation of vertebral symmetry in 2D and in 3D, did not yield variability as low as the mid-wall lines or posterior tangents, but were still comparable to the superior and inferior tangents, i.e. to the standard Cobb angle measurements. It can be therefore concluded that for manual measurements, the evaluation of SVI in MR images should be based on the inclination of vertebral body walls and not vertebral endplates, while for computerized measurements, the evaluation of the symmetry of vertebral anatomical structures is in its current application form not the best choice to evaluate SVI in MR images.

Acknowledgments This work has been supported by the Slovenian Research Agency under grants P2-0232, J7-2264, L2-7381, and L2-2023. The authors thank R. Vengust (University Medical Centre Ljubljana, Slovenia) and D. Štern (University of Ljubljana, Slovenia) for performing manual measurements.

References

1. Singer, K., Edmondston, S., Day, R., Breidahl, W.: Computer-assisted curvature assessment and Cobb angle determination of the thoracic kyphosis: an in vivo and in vitro comparison. Spine **19**(12), 1381–1384 (1994)
2. Chernukha, K., Daffner, R., Reigel, D.: Lumbar lordosis measurement: a new method versus Cobb technique. Spine **23**(1), 74–79 (1998)
3. Harrison, D., Cailliet, R., Janik, T., Troyanovich, S., Harrison, D., Holland, B.: Elliptical modeling of the sagittal lumbar lordosis and segmental rotation angles as a method to discriminate between normal and low back pain subjects. J. Spinal Disord. **11**(5), 430–439 (1998)
4. Chen, Y.L.: Vertebral centroid measurement of lumbar lordosis compared with the Cobb technique. Spine **24**(17), 1786–1790 (1999)
5. Cobb, J.: Outline for the study of scoliosis. Am. Acad. Orthop. Surg. Instr. Course Lectur. **5**, 261–275 (1948)
6. Gore, D., Sepic, S., Gardner, G.: Roentgenographic findings of the cervical spine in asymptomatic people. Spine **11**(6), 521–524 (1986)
7. Harrison, D., Janik, T., Troyanovich, S., Holland, B.: Comparisons of lordotic cervical spine curvatures to a theoretical ideal model of the static sagittal cervical spine. Spine **21**(6), 667–675 (1996)
8. Schuler, T., Subach, B., Branch, C., Foley, K., Burkus, J.: Lumbar spine study group: segmental lumbar lordosis: manual versus computer-assisted measurement using seven different techniques. J. Spinal Disord. Tech. **17**(5), 372–379 (2004)
9. Polly, D., Kilkelly, F., McHale, K., Asplund, L., Mulligan, M., Chang, A.: Measurement of lumbar lordosis: evaluation of intraobserver, interobserver, and technique variability. Spine **21**(13), 1530–1535 (1996)
10. Goh, S., Price, R., Leedman, P., Singer, K.: A comparison of three methods for measuring thoracic kyphosis: implications for clinical studies. Rheumatology **39**(3), 310–315 (2000)
11. Mac-Thiong, J.M., Labelle, H., Charlebois, M., Huot, M.P., de Guise, J.: Sagittal plane analysis of the spine and pelvis in adolescent idiopathic scoliosis according to the coronal curve type. Spine **28**(13), 1404–1409 (2003)

12. Stagnara, P., De Mauroy, J., Dran, G., Gonon, G., Costanzo, G., Dimnet, J., Pasquet, A.: Reciprocal angulation of vertebral bodies in a sagittal plane: approach to references for the evaluation of kyphosis and lordosis. Spine 7(4), 335–342 (1982)
13. Bernhardt, M., Bridwell, K.: Segmental analysis of the sagittal plane alignment of the normal thoracic and lumbar spines and thoracolumbar junction. Spine 14(7), 717–721 (1989)
14. Korovessis, P., Stamatakis, M., Baikousis, A.: Reciprocal angulation of vertebral bodies in the sagittal plane in an asymptomatic Greek population. Spine 23(6), 700–704 (1998)
15. Street, J., Lenehan, B., Albietz, J., Bishop, P., Dvorak, M., Fisher, C.: Spine Trauma Study Group: Intraobserver and interobserver reliabilty of measures of kyphosis in thoracolumbar fractures. Spine J. 9(6), 464–469 (2009)
16. Birchall, D., Hughes, D., Hindle, J., Robinson, L., Williamson, J.: Measurement of vertebral rotation in adolescent idiopathic scoliosis using three-dimensional magnetic resonance imaging. Spine 22(20), 2403–2407 (1997)
17. Haughton, V., Rogers, B., Meyerand, E., Resnick, D.: Measuring the axial rotation of lumbar vertebrae in vivo with MR imaging. Am. J. Neuroradiol. 23(7), 1110–1116 (2002)
18. Rogers, B., Haughton, V., Arfanakis, K., Meyerand, M.: Application of image registration to measurement of intervertebral rotation in the lumbar spine. Magn. Reson. Med. 48(6), 1072–1075 (2002)
19. Birchall, D., Hughes, D., Gregson, B., Williamson, B.: Demonstration of vertebral and disc mechanical torsion in adolescent idiopathic scoliosis using three-dimensional MR imaging. Eur. Spine J. 14(2), 123–129 (2005)
20. Kouwenhoven, J.W., Bartels, L., Vincken, K., Viergever, M., Verbout, A., Delhaas, T., Castelein, R.: The relation between organ anatomy and pre-existent vertebral rotation in the normal spine: magnetic resonance imaging study in humans with situs inversus totalis. Spine 32(10), 1123–1128 (2007)
21. Vrtovec, T., Pernuš, F., Likar, B.: Determination of axial vertebral rotation in MR images: comparison of four manual and a computerized method. Eur. Spine J. 19(5), 774–781 (2010)
22. Vrtovec, T., Likar, B., Pernuš, F.: Manual and computerized measurement of coronal vertebral inclination in MRI images: a pilot study. Clin. Radiol. 68(8), 807–814 (2013)
23. Vrtovec, T., Pernuš, F., Likar, B.: A symmetry-based method for the determination of vertebral rotation in 3D Lecture Notes in Computer Science. Lecture Notes in Computer Science, pp. 942–950. Springer, Berlin (2008)
24. Vrtovec, T., Likar, B., Pernuš, F.: Manual and computerized measurement of sagittal vertebral inclination in computed tomography images. Spine 36(13), E875–E881 (2011)
25. Vrtovec, T., Vengust, R., Likar, B., Pernuš, F.: Analysis of four manual and a computerized method for measuring axial vertebral rotation in computed tomography images. Spine 35(12), E535–E541 (2010)

Eigenspine: Eigenvector Analysis of Spinal Deformities in Idiopathic Scoliosis

Daniel Forsberg, Claes Lundström, Mats Andersson and Hans Knutsson

Abstract In this paper, we propose the concept of eigenspine, a data analysis scheme useful for quantifying the linear correlation between different measures relevant for describing spinal deformities associated with spinal diseases, such as idiopathic scoliosis. The proposed concept builds upon the use of principal component analysis (PCA) and canonical correlation analysis (CCA), where PCA is used to reduce the number of dimensions in the measurement space, thereby providing a regularization of the measurements, and where CCA is used to determine the linear dependence between pair-wise combinations of the different measures. To demonstrate the usefulness of the eigenspine concept, the measures describing position and rotation of the lumbar and the thoracic vertebrae of 22 patients suffering from idiopathic scoliosis were analyzed. The analysis showed that the strongest linear relationship is found between the anterior-posterior displacement and the sagittal rotation of the vertebrae, and that a somewhat weaker but still strong correlation is found between the lateral displacement and the frontal rotation of the vertebrae. These results are well in-line

D. Forsberg (✉) · C. Lundström · M. Andersson · H. Knutsson
Center for Medical Image Science and Visualization, Linköping University,
Linköping, Sweden
e-mail: daniel.forsberg@sectra.se

M. Andersson
e-mail: mats.x.andersson@liu.se

H. Knutsson
e-mail: hans.knutsson@liu.se

M. Andersson · H. Knutsson
Department of Biomedical Engineering, Linköping University, Linköping, Sweden

C. Lundström
e-mail: claes.lundstrom@sectra.se

D. Forsberg · C. Lundström
Sectra, Linköping, Sweden

J. Yao et al. (eds.), *Computational Methods and Clinical Applications*
for Spine Imaging, Lecture Notes in Computational Vision and Biomechanics 17,
DOI: 10.1007/978-3-319-07269-2_11, © Springer International Publishing Switzerland 2014

with the general understanding of idiopathic scoliosis. Noteworthy though is that the obtained results from the analysis further proposes axial vertebral rotation as a differentiating measure when characterizing idiopathic scoliosis. Apart from analyzing pair-wise linear correlations between different measures, the method is believed to be suitable for finding a maximally descriptive low-dimensional combination of measures describing spinal deformities in idiopathic scoliosis.

1 Introduction

Idiopathic scoliosis is a disease affecting the spine by causing an excessive lateral curvature, as observed in the frontal plane, and is estimated to have a prevalence rate of 2–3 % for the age group 10–16 years old [13, 18]. The disease is typically categorized according to curvature type (C- or S-like), location of the primary curvature (thoracic, lumbar or thoracolumbar) and age of onset (infantile, juvenile, adolescent or adult). The choice of treatment, i.e. bracing or surgery, is dependent on a number of factors, which include age of onset, gender, skeletal maturity, the Cobb angle and the estimated progression rate. Especially the Cobb angle plays an important role in deciding which treatment to use. The Cobb angle is defined as the angle between two lines drawn parallel to the superior endplate of the superior end vertebra and parallel to the inferior endplate of the inferior end vertebra as observed in an anterior-posterior radiograph [1]. However, although an established measure, the Cobb angle measures a 2D projection of what is actually a 3D deformity, and, therefore, the relevance of using the Cobb angle alone for assessment of the spinal deformity of a scoliotic curvature can be questioned. To this end, a number of other methods for assessing spinal deformity have been developed, including both manual and computerized methods. Examples include methods for axial vertebral rotation measurements [11, 17], based on either 2D or 3D data, and methods for estimating both the position and the rotation of each vertebra [2, 5, 16].

Apart from developing methods that can provide a more accurate 3D description of the spinal deformity of a scoliotic curvature, there is also a need to analyze how different measures describing spinal deformities relate to each other and to the clinical outcome [4, 6, 15]. This is important in order to classify various sub-types of idiopathic scoliosis and to determine if different treatments are suitable for the different sub-types of idiopathic scoliosis. Examples of this kind of work are found in [3, 7, 14], where they apply clustering algorithms to the measures derived from the EOS system [2], in order to identify various sub-types of idiopathic scoliosis. However, there has been limited amount of work performed, aimed at analyzing the relation between different measures relevant for assessing spinal deformities. To this end, we present the concept of eigenspine, a data analysis scheme for analyzing the linear correlation between different measures relevant for describing spinal deformities.

2 Eigenspine

The proposed data analysis scheme is based on a combination of principal component analysis (PCA) and canonical correlation analysis (CCA), where PCA is used to reduce the number of dimensions in the measurement space, i.e. a regularization, and CCA is used to determine the linear dependence between pair-wise combinations of the different measures. Although, in this work, the proposed scheme is primarily employed to analyze the linear dependence between various measures, the long-term goal of the analysis is to determine which measures, or combination of measures, that are significant for describing and assessing a scoliotic curvature and, thus, providing an approach for creating a classification scheme similar to the ones that are typically used, e.g. King and Lenke [10, 12], but in this case relying on a 3D description of the deformity, instead of merely using 2D projections of a 3D deformity.

2.1 PCA and CCA

PCA and CCA are two standard techniques for exploring data and is typically applied in unsupervised learning. For the sake of completeness, we will briefly introduce the two methods. Let X denote a data matrix

$$X = \begin{bmatrix} \mathbf{x}_1 & \mathbf{x}_2 & \cdots & \mathbf{x}_n \end{bmatrix}, \tag{1}$$

where

$$\mathbf{x}_i = \begin{bmatrix} x_1 & x_2 & \cdots & x_p \end{bmatrix}^T, \tag{2}$$

i.e. X contains n measurements of p variables. Compute the covariance matrix $\mathbf{C}_X$ as

$$\mathbf{C}_X \approx \frac{1}{n-1}(X - \bar{X})(X - \bar{X})^T, \tag{3}$$

Define similarly a data matrix Y.

For PCA, a linear transform W is estimated such that the variance of the components of $Z = W^T X$ is maximized under the constraint that the components $\mathbf{w}_i$ of W are orthogonal, i.e. the components of Z are uncorrelated and $\mathbf{C}_Z = W^T \mathbf{C}_X W$ is diagonal. In CCA, two linear transforms, W_X and W_Y, are estimated such that the correlation ρ_i between the reduced variables (canonical variates) of $W_{X,i}^T X$ and $W_{Y,i}^T Y$, have been maximized and that the different components of $W_{X,i}^T X$ and $W_{Y,i}^T Y$ are uncorrelated with respect to each other. Note that for CCA, the data matrices X and Y are not required to have the same number of variables, therefore the number of canonical variates will correspond to the smallest number of variables provided by either X or Y. Estimating the linear transforms W in PCA, and W_X and W_Y in CCA are done solving an eigenvector problem, hence, the term eigenspine.

An interesting aspect of CCA is its relation with mutual information (MI). As shown by [9], the mutual information between X and Y can be estimated as the sum of the mutual information of the reduced variables, given that their statistical dependence is limited to correlation. For normally distributed variables, this relation is given as

$$\text{MI}(X, Y) = \frac{1}{2} \sum_i \log_2 \left(\frac{1}{(1 - \rho_i^2)} \right). \tag{4}$$

This follows from considering a continuous random variable $\mathbf{x}$ with the differential entropy defined as

$$h(\mathbf{x}) = - \int_{\mathbb{R}^N} p(\mathbf{x}) \log_2 (p(\mathbf{x})) \, d\mathbf{x}, \tag{5}$$

where $p(\mathbf{x})$ is the probability density function of $\mathbf{x}$. Consider similarly a continuous random variable $\mathbf{y}$, then it can be shown that

$$\text{MI}(\mathbf{x}, \mathbf{y}) = h(\mathbf{x}) + h(\mathbf{y}) - h(\mathbf{x}, \mathbf{y}) = \int_{\mathbb{R}^M} \int_{\mathbb{R}^N} p(\mathbf{x}, \mathbf{y}) \log_2 \left(\frac{p(\mathbf{x}, \mathbf{y})}{p(\mathbf{x}) p(\mathbf{y})} \right) d\mathbf{x} d\mathbf{y}. \tag{6}$$

Further, consider a Gaussian distributed variable $\mathbf{z}$, for which the differential entropy is given as

$$h(\mathbf{z}) = \frac{1}{2} \log_2 \left((2\pi e)^N |\mathbf{C}| \right), \tag{7}$$

where $\mathbf{C}$ is the covariance matrix of $\mathbf{z}$. In the case of two N-dimensional variables, then (6) becomes

$$\text{MI}(\mathbf{x}, \mathbf{y}) = \frac{1}{2} \log_2 \left(\frac{|\mathbf{C}_{xx}||\mathbf{C}_{yy}|}{\mathbf{C}} \right), \tag{8}$$

where

$$\mathbf{C} = \begin{bmatrix} \mathbf{C}_{xx} & \mathbf{C}_{xy} \\ \mathbf{C}_{yx} & \mathbf{C}_{yy} \end{bmatrix}. \tag{9}$$

For two one-dimensional Gaussian distributed variables, (8) reduces to

$$\text{MI}(x, y) = \frac{1}{2} \log_2 \left(\frac{\sigma_x^2 \sigma_y^2}{\sigma_x^2 \sigma_y^2 - \sigma_{xy}^2} \right) = \frac{1}{2} \log_2 \left(\frac{1}{1 - \rho_{xy}^2} \right), \tag{10}$$

where σ_x^2 and σ_y^2 are the variances of x and y, σ_{xy}^2 is the covariance of x and y and ρ_{xy} is the correlation between x and y. Given that information is additive, for statistically independent variables, and that the canonical variates are uncorrelated, i.e. $\mathbf{W}_{X,i}^T \mathbf{X}$ and $\mathbf{W}_{Y,i}^T \mathbf{Y}$, hence, the mutual information between $\mathbf{X}$ and $\mathbf{Y}$ is the sum of the mutual information between the variates.

Note that using the log-function with the base 2 provides an MI measure defined in bits. This measure will be employed in the subsequent analysis for quantifying the dependence between different measures.

3 Experiments

To demonstrate the use of the data analysis scheme, measurements of the position and the orientation of the vertebrae for a number of patients were analyzed to determine which of these measures that have the strongest linear dependence.

3.1 Image Data

Image data from 22 patients (19 female and three male) were retrospectively gathered and extracted from the local picture archiving and communications system. The only criteria for inclusion was that the patient suffered from idiopathic scoliosis and that the CT data had a resolution higher than $1 \times 1 \times 1\,\text{mm}^3$. The data sets depicted all lumbar and thoracic vertebrae, i.e. 17 vertebrae per patient. The requirement on the resolution was needed in order to be able to distinguish adjacent vertebrae in the subsequently applied method for obtaining the position and rotation of each vertebra. The patients had an average age of 16.0 ± 3.1 years at the time of their respective examinations and an average Cobb angle of $60.4° \pm 9.6$ (standing position). Most patients were classified has having a scoliosis of Lenke type 3C or 4C.

The images were captured as a part of the standard routine for pre-operational planning and they were anonymized before being exported by clinical staff. Note that for patients of similar age as included in this retrospective study, it is often questionable whether a CT scan is appropriate or not, due to the exposure to radiation. However, at the local hospital there is a protocol in place for acquiring low-dose CT examinations with maintained image quality, targeted towards examinations of the spine. With the use of this protocol, the radiation dose is approximately 0.4 mSv. More on this can be found in [8].

3.2 Curvature Measures

Each data set was processed with the method presented in [5], which is based on the following steps; *extraction of the spinal canal centerline*, *disc detection*, *vertebra centerpoint estimation* and *vertebra rotation estimation*. A graphical overview of the method is provided in Fig. 1. In [5], the method was shown to have a variability, when compared with manual measurements, that is on par with the inter-observer variability for measuring the axial vertebral rotation. This was supported by Bland-

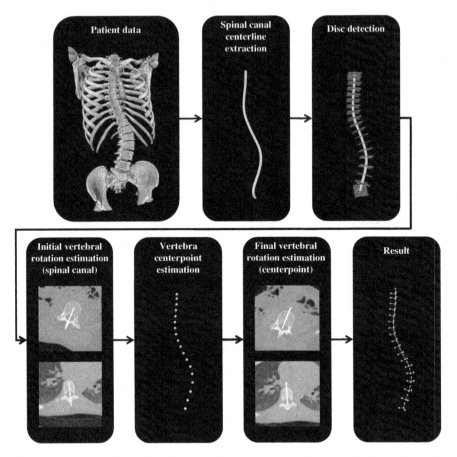

Fig. 1 An overview of the method for automatic measurements of the pose of each vertebra in the spine

Altman plots and high values of the intraclass correlation coefficient, thus, showing that the method can be used as a replacement for manual measurements.

The method estimates, for each vertebra, the position $[x, y, z]$ and the rotation matrix R, from which the rotation angles $[\theta_X, \theta_Y, \theta_Z]$ can be derived. The rotation angles were computed as the Euler angles (using a fixed world frame) of the rotation matrix R. Note the order of the rotational angles, $R = R_Z(\theta_Z)R_Y(\theta_Y)R_X(\theta_X)$. θ_Z corresponds to axial vertebral rotation, θ_Y to frontal rotation and θ_X to sagittal rotation. The standard DICOM patient coordinate system was employed to define the orientation of $[x, y, z]$, i.e. x increases from right to left, y from anterior to posterior and z from inferior to superior.

3.3 Curvature Analysis

In the data analysis, the curves of each measure, apart from the z-coordinates, for the entire spine were analyzed. The estimated z-coordinates were neglected and the vertebrae indexes were set to define the dimensions of the measurements per curve, i.e. each measure was embedded into a 17 dimensional space. Note that the z-coordinates were neglected, since the analysis is performed considering all measurements for a specific measure and patient simultaneously. Furthermore, the x- and y-coordinates of all vertebrae were translated in order to have the common starting point $(0, 0)$ for all L5 vertebrae. Each curve ensemble was then processed with PCA to find its principal components. After the PCA, CCA was applied on the measures projected onto the subspace spanned by the largest PCA eigenvectors of each measure. The CCA was applied to analyze the dependence between all pair-wise combinations of the different measures.

A reasonable question at this point is why CCA is not applied directly on the estimated measures. The reason for this is two-fold. First, due to the large number of variables (17 vertebrae) compared to the low number of observations (22 patients), which can cause singularities in the computations of the CCA, a dimension reduction was called for. Second, using CCA directly is likely to generate an overfitting, i.e. it can find correlations related more to noise in the signal than to the relevant variations in the signal, hence, smoothing or a regularization was called for. Both of these requirements can be met by performing a PCA and projecting the data onto the subspace spanned by the eigenvectors.

4 Results

In the conducted experiments, PCA was applied to each estimated measure, apart from the z-coordinates, over all patients, followed by a CCA on each pair-wise combination of the measures. From the estimated eigenvalues, the eigenvectors, corresponding to at least 99 % of the variance in the data, were extracted. This meant for instance that the variance in x-coordinates could be reduced to four eigenvectors, whereas the curves of θ_X required six eigenvectors. Figure 2 depicts the measurements over all measures and patients, and Fig. 3 the extracted eigenvectors for each measure. Figure 4 depicts the reconstruction error between the original curves and the curves projected onto the subspace of the extracted eigenvectors.

The CCA was applied onto every pair-wise combination of the measures, where the measures were projected onto the subspace spanned by the extracted eigenvectors from the PCA. This was done to find dependencies between the different measures. Table 1 provides the obtained canonical correlations of all pair-wise CCAs along with corresponding MI estimates. Note the difference in number of canonical correlation coefficients between the different pair-wise comparisons, which is due to the different number of extracted eigenvectors per measure.

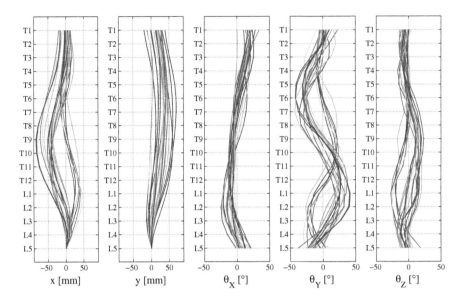

Fig. 2 All estimated measurements for all measures and all patients are depicted

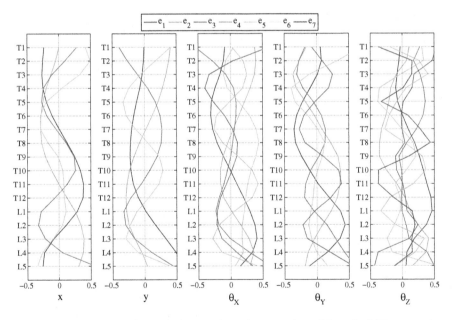

Fig. 3 Eigenvectors belonging to the largest eigenvalues as estimated from the PCA, accounting for at least 99 % of the variance in the data

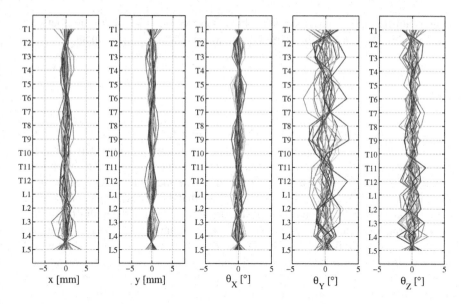

Fig. 4 Reconstruction error as given by the difference between the original curves and the curves projected onto the subspace of the eigenvectors accounting for 99 % of the variance in the data

Table 1 Canonical correlations and MI as obtained from the pair-wise CCA, sorted according to estimated MI

	ρ_1	ρ_2	ρ_3	ρ_4	ρ_5	ρ_6	MI
$y - \theta_X$	1.00	0.99	0.99	0.97			13.01
$x - \theta_Y$	1.00	0.99	0.99	0.80			10.69
$\theta_Y - \theta_Z$	0.99	0.96	0.92	0.81	0.39		7.10
$x - \theta_Z$	0.99	0.94	0.90	0.67			6.09
$\theta_X - \theta_Z$	0.90	0.87	0.72	0.70	0.49	0.15	3.46
$\theta_X - \theta_Y$	0.86	0.78	0.75	0.60	0.35		2.67
$y - \theta_Z$	0.88	0.70	0.53	0.36			1.88
$x - \theta_X$	0.78	0.74	0.53	0.43			1.65
$y - \theta_Y$	0.82	0.72	0.48	0.13			1.55
$x - y$	0.71	0.49	0.45	0.16			0.90

Here ρ_i denotes the correlation between the canonical variates, e.g. between $W_{X,i}^T X_y$ and $W_{Y,i}^T Y_{\theta_X}$ and where $\rho_i \geq \rho_{i+1}$. The MI-values are estimated in accordance with (4)

The results show that the strongest linear dependence exists between the y-coordinates and θ_X. A somewhat weaker but still obvious dependence is found between the x-coordinates and θ_Y. A second group of linear relationships, however, substantially weaker than the first two, is found between θ_Y and θ_Z, and between x and θ_Z. Or, as expressed in anatomical terms, the anterior-posterior displacement of the vertebral body is highly correlated with the sagittal rotation of the same. In addition, lateral displacement and frontal rotation of the vertebrae are highly correlated. Substantially weaker but still obvious correlations are also found between axial vertebral rotation and both frontal rotation and lateral displacement.

5 Discussion

This paper has presented the concept of eigenspine, a data analysis scheme for determining the relationship between different measures related to spinal deformity. The potential usage of the method has been exemplified by analyzing the dependence between different measures describing spinal deformities. The results of the combined PCA and CCA analysis show, for example, that the strongest linear dependencies are found between the anterior-posterior displacement and sagittal rotation of the vertebral body and between the lateral displacement and frontal rotation of the vertebrae. That there is a strong linear dependence between these measures is well in-line with what would be expected and what is previously known. However, more interesting conclusions can be drawn, once the different pair-wise linear dependencies are compared, since this analysis can indicate which measures that are the most relevant for describing a scoliotic curvature.

For instance, the fact that the strongest linear relationships exist between the pair-wise measures $y - \theta_X$ and $x - \theta_Y$ indicates that to describe a scoliotic curvature it suffices to either measure the sagittal rotation θ_X and the frontal rotation θ_Y or the lateral and the anterior-posterior displacements x and y. Given that there is some linear relationship between axial vertebral rotation θ_Z and both frontal rotation θ_Y and lateral displacement x, but that it is substantially weaker then the two primary linear correlations, a tentative hypothesis would be that axial vertebral rotation θ_Z is a differentiating factor when describing a scoliotic curvature. An understanding that adds support to the recent interest in quantifying the axial vertebral rotation when assessing idiopathic scoliosis. This further indicates that the classification systems by King and by Lenke [10, 12], are insufficient to fully differentiate between different types of scoliosis, since the axial vertebral rotation is not included in their respective classification systems. However, given the limited number of included patients, further analysis including more patients is called for, before any conclusions can be made.

It is important to point out that the obtained quantification of the linear dependencies between all pair-wise combinations of measures via the computed MI, relies on the assumption of normal distributions for all included variables. An assumption that is questionable whether it holds, and, thus, needs further analysis.

Further, it can be noted that the data analysis scheme has been employed to measures based upon a method for estimating the pose of each vertebra as derived from CT data. However, the eigenspine concept is not limited to these measures or the used method, but could be readily applied to other measurements obtained with e.g. the EOS system. An analysis based upon the data employed in [3, 7, 14] would be interesting to pursue in order to further quantify the relation between different measures, since the patient groups employed therein are rather large. Another interesting future aspect would be to include other measures, e.g. measures related to the deformation that the vertebral bodies undergo during the progression of the scoliotic curvature.

In this work, only the linear correlation between pair-wise combinations of measures have been analyzed. However, using CCA we believe it would be possible to extend this analysis further, but instead analyzing information content for any number of combined measures by employing autocorrelation. This could be useful to determine a maximally descriptive low-dimensional combination of measures describing spinal deformities in idiopathic scoliosis, and thereby providing means to better relate treatment and outcome of different types of idiopathic scoliosis, which would be a significant clinical outcome.

Acknowledgments The authors would like to thank L. Vavruch and H. Tropp at the Department of Clinical and Experimental Medicine, Linköping University, Sweden, for valuable input in discussions regarding idiopathic scoliosis and for assistance in collecting the used image data. This work was funded by the Swedish Research Council (grant 2007-4786) and the Swedish Foundation for Strategic Research (grant SM10-0022).

References

1. Cobb, R., Cobb, R.: Outline for study of scoliosis. Am. Acad. Orthop. Surg. Instr. Course Lect. **5**, 261–275 (1948)
2. Dubousset, J., Charpak, G., Dorion, I., Skalli, W., Lavaste, F., Deguise, J., Kalifa, G., Ferey, S.: A new 2D and 3D imaging approach to musculoskeletal physiology and pathology with low-dose radiation and the standing position: the EOS system. Bulletin de l'Academie nationale de medecine **189**(2), 287 (2005)
3. Duong, L., Cheriet, F., Labelle, H.: Three-dimensional classification of spinal deformities using fuzzy clustering. Spine **31**(8), 923–930 (2006)
4. Easwar, T., Hong, J., Yang, J., Suh, S., Modi, H.: Does lateral vertebral translation correspond to Cobb angle and relate in the same way to axial vertebral rotation and rib hump index? A radiographic analysis on idiopathic scoliosis. Eur. Spine J. **20**(7), 1095–1105 (2011)
5. Forsberg, D., Lundström, C., Andersson, M., Vavruch, L., Tropp, H., Knutsson, H.: Fully automatic measurements of axial vertebral rotation for assessment of spinal deformity in idiopathic scoliosis. Phys. Med. Biol. **58**(6), 1775–1787 (2013)
6. Hong, J.Y., Suh, S.W., Easwar, T.R., Modi, H.N., Yang, J.H., Park, J.H.: Evaluation of the three-dimensional deformities in scoliosis surgery with computed tomography: efficacy and relationship with clinical outcomes. Spine **36**(19), E1259–E1265 (2011)
7. Kadoury, S., Labelle, H.: Classification of three-dimensional thoracic deformities in adolescent idiopathic scoliosis from a multivariate analysis. Eur. Spine J. **21**(1), 40–49 (2012)
8. Kalra, M.K., Quick, P., Singh, S., Sandborg, M., Persson, A.: Whole spine CT for evaluation of scoliosis in children: feasibility of sub-millisievert scanning protocol. Acta Radiologica **54**(2), 226–230 (2013)
9. Kay, J.: Feature discovery under contextual supervision using mutual information. In: International Joint Conference on Neural Networks, 1992. IJCNN, vol. 4, pp. 79–84 IEEE (1992)
10. King, H.A., Moe, J.H., Bradford, D.S., Winter, R.B.: The selection of fusion levels in thoracic idiopathic scoliosis. J. Bone Joint Surg. Am. **65**(9), 1302–1313 (1983)
11. Lam, G., Hill, D., Le, L., Raso, J., Lou, E.: Vertebral rotation measurement: a summary and comparison of common radiographic and CT methods. Scoliosis **3**(1), 16 (2008)

12. Lenke, L.G., Betz, R.R., Harms, J., Bridwell, K.H., Clements, D.H., Lowe, T.G., Blanke, K.: Adolescent idiopathic scoliosis a new classification to determine extent of spinal arthrodesis. J. Bone Joint Surg. **83**(8), 1169–1181 (2001)
13. Reamy, B.V., Slakey, J.B.: Adolescent idiopathic scoliosis: review and current concepts. Am. Fam. Phys. **64**(1), 111–117 (2001)
14. Sangole, A.P., Aubin, C.E., Labelle, H., Stokes, I.A.F., Lenke, L.G., Jackson, R., Newton, P.: Three-dimensional classification of thoracic scoliotic curves. Spine **34**(1), 91–99 (2008)
15. Schwab, F.J., Smith, V.A., Biserni, M., Gamez, L., Farcy, J.P.C., Pagala, M.: Adult scoliosis: a quantitative radiographic and clinical analysis. Spine **27**(4), 387–392 (2002)
16. Vrtovec, T.: Modality-independent Determination of Vertebral Position and Rotation in 3D. Medical Imaging and Augmented Reality, pp. 89–97. Springer, Berlin (2008)
17. Vrtovec, T., Pernuš, F., Likar, B.: A review of methods for quantitative evaluation of axial vertebral rotation. Eur. Spine J. **18**, 1079–1090 (2009)
18. Weinstein, S.L., Dolan, L.A., Cheng, J.C., Danielsson, A., Morcuende, J.A.: Adolescent idiopathic scoliosis. Lancet **371**(9623), 1527–1537 (2008)

Quantitative Monitoring of Syndesmophyte Growth in Ankylosing Spondylitis Using Computed Tomography

Sovira Tan, Jianhua Yao, Lawrence Yao and Michael M. Ward

Abstract Ankylosing Spondylitis, an inflammatory disease affecting mainly the spine, can be characterized by abnormal bone formation (syndesmophytes) along the margins of the intervertebral disk. Monitoring syndesmophytes evolution is challenging because of their slow growth rate, a problem compounded by the use of radiography and qualitative rating systems. To improve sensitivity to change, we designed a computer algorithm that fully quantifies syndesmophyte volume using the 3D imaging capabilities of computed tomography. The reliability of the algorithm was assessed by comparing the results obtained from 2 scans performed on the same day in 9 patients. A longitudinal study on 20 patients suggests that the method will benefit longitudinal clinical studies of syndesmophyte development and growth. After one year, the 3D algorithm showed an increase in syndesmophyte volume in 75 % of patients, while radiography showed an increase in only 15 % of patients.

1 Introduction

Ankylosing Spondylitis (AS) is an uncommon inflammatory arthritis affecting primarily the spine. Progression of AS is characterized by abnormal bone (syndesmophytes) formation along the margins of inter-vertebral disk spaces (IDS). Syndesmophytes cause irreversible and progressive structural damage, and over decades, can lead to spinal fusion [1]. Monitoring syndesmophyte evolution is essential for many

S. Tan (✉) · M. M. Ward
National Institute of Arthritis and Musculoskeletal and Skin Diseases,
National Institutes of Health, Bethesda, MD 20892, USA
e-mail: tanso@mail.nih.gov

J. Yao · L. Yao
Radiology and Imaging Sciences, Clinical Center, National Institutes of Health,
Bethesda, MD 20892, USA
e-mail: jyao@cc.nih.gov

J. Yao et al. (eds.), *Computational Methods and Clinical Applications*
for Spine Imaging, Lecture Notes in Computational Vision and Biomechanics 17,
DOI: 10.1007/978-3-319-07269-2_12, © Springer International Publishing Switzerland 2014

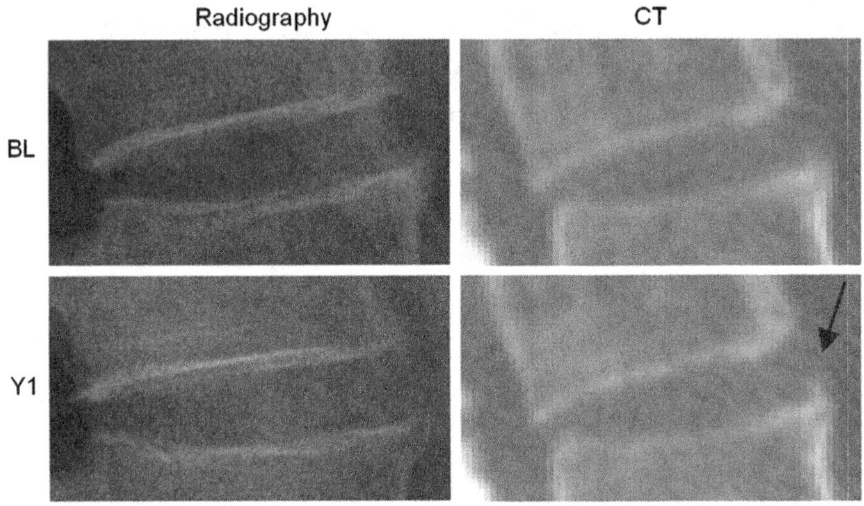

Radiography   CT

Fig. 1 Example of syndesmophyte growth from baseline (BL) to year 1 (Y1) visible on CT reformations but not on radiographs

clinical studies of AS. Newly available treatmentsneed to be tested to determine if they slow rates of syndesmophyte growth [2]. Considerable research has been aimed at understanding the molecular mechanisms of bone formation in AS, and the correlation between syndesmophyte growth and specific gene expression [3, 4]. Unfortunately, such studies have been hampered by the fact the current standard for assessing syndesmophyte growth, the visual examination of radiographs, has very poor sensitivity to change. This low sensitivity to change is not only a reflection of the slow growth rate of syndesmophytes. It is also caused by the limitations of radiography, which projects 3D objects onto 2D images with attendant losses of spatial information and ambiguities in density caused by superimposition. Moreover, the use of coarse semi-quantitative reading systems also severely limits sensitivity to change [5, 6]. Figure 1 shows an example of syndesmophyte growth visible on reformatted CT but not radiography.

To overcome the limitations of radiographic methods, we designed a computer algorithm that quantitatively measures syndesmophyte volumes in the 3D space of CT scans [7, 8].

2 The Algorithm

The complete algorithm, summarized in Fig. 2, has of three main parts. First, vertebral bodies are segmented using a 3D multi-stage level set method. Triangular meshes representing the surfaces of the segmentations are made. The 3D surfaces

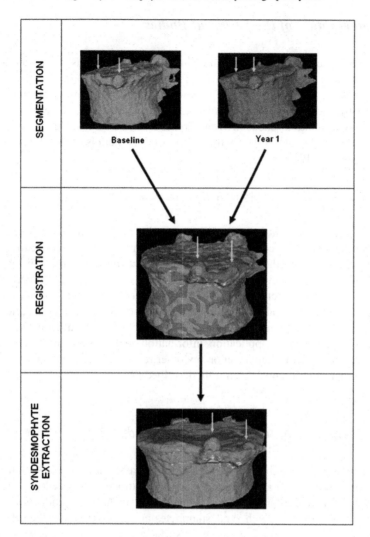

Fig. 2 Overview of the complete algorithm

shown in Fig. 2 are triangular meshes obtained from our segmentation results. The vertebral surfaces of corresponding vertebrae are then registered. The purpose of the registration is to extract the syndesmophytes of both vertebrae using the same reference level. Syndesmophytes are cut from the vertebral body using the end plate's ridgeline as the reference level.

2.1 Segmentation of the Vertebral Bodies

Many image processing segmentation techniques have previously been applied to the extraction of vertebral bodies in CT [9–11]. For our algorithm, we chose to use level sets for their flexibility [12]. Flexibility is essential in our application as syndesmophytes can deform the normal vertebral structure in unexpected ways. Level sets are evolving contours encoded as the zero level set of a distance function $\psi\,(\vec{x}, t)$. Points that verify $\psi\,(\vec{x}, t) = 0$ form the contour. The contour is made to evolve using equations such as [13]:

$$\frac{d\psi}{dt} = \alpha g\,(\vec{x})\,c\,|\nabla\psi| + \beta g\,(\vec{x})\,\kappa\,|\nabla\psi| + \gamma\,\nabla g\,(\vec{x})\,\nabla\psi. \tag{1}$$

The three terms on the right-hand side of the equation respectively control the expansion or contraction of the contour (velocity c), the smoothness of the contour using the mean curvature κ and the adherence of the contour to the boundary of the object to be segmented. The parameters α, β and γ allow the user to weight the importance of each term. The spatial function $g\,(\vec{x})$, often called speed function, is derived from the images to be segmented and contains information about the objects' boundaries. The design of the speed function is crucial for the success of the segmentation. Depending on the specific needs of the application, information on the object's boundary can be based on image gradient, Laplacian or any other relevant feature. Details about our level set implementation have been fully described [7].

2.2 Segmentation of the Vertebral Body Ridgelines

The segmentation of vertebral body ridgelines is a preliminary step to both the registration stage (Sect. 2.3) and the syndesmophyte extraction stage (Sect. 2.4). The vertebral body ridgelines provide the landmarks that aid the registration process and the reference level from which syndesmophytes are cut. We extract the ridgelines from the triangular meshes representing the surfaces of the vertebrae using the same level set as Eq. 1, but transposed from the Cartesian domain of rectangular grids to the domain of a surface mesh. The most important adjustment is to design a suitable speed function. While in the usual image grids of CT scans the relevant features are grey level gradients, on a surface mesh, the useful features are curvature measures (the vertebral body surface is more curved at the ridgelines than on the end plates). The curvature measure we used is curvedness (C) [14]:

$$C = \sqrt{\frac{\kappa_1^2 + \kappa_2^2}{2}} \tag{2}$$

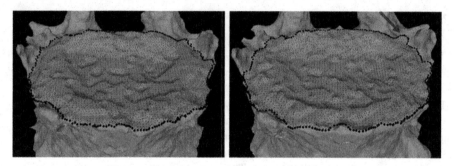

Fig. 3 End plate (*red*) and ridgeline (*black*) segmentation at baseline (*left*) and year 1 (*right*)

where κ_1 and κ_2 are the principal curvatures. The speed function ensures that the level set contour expands in the center of the end plates and stops at the ridgelines. The most complete description of the mesh level set can be found in [7].

Figure 3 shows an example of ridgeline segmentation at baseline and year 1. Bone above the ridgeline will be labeled as syndesmophyte. Some small differences between the 2 ridgelines are visible (arrow). Although the difference can seem minor, it can lead to differences in syndesmophyte volume measurements. Such differences would not be due to real syndesmophyte growth. Because real growth may be small, it is important to reduce the error coming from ridgeline discrepancies. That is the motivation behind the next step, registration, which aligns the 2 vertebral surfaces so that only one of the ridgelines needs to be used as the reference level from which to cut syndesmophytes.

2.3 Vertebral Body Registration

We used the iterative closest point (ICP) algorithm to register the surfaces of the vertebrae segmented at baseline and year 1. Given 2 sets of points, the ICP algorithm finds the rigid transformation that minimizes the mean square distance between them [15]. We added landmark matching to address the problem of entrapment in local minima. Our ICP algorithm is performed successively on the ridgelines, end plates and the complete surface, the result of each stage serving as the initialization for the following stage [16]. An example of registration results is shown in Fig. 2 (middle). The registration step makes the algorithm robust to small errors in ridgeline segmentation.

2.4 Syndesmophyte Segmentation

Once corresponding pairs of vertebrae are registered, syndesmophytes can be cut from the vertebral bodies using the ridgeline of either the baseline (our choice in the present work) or year 1 vertebra. The algorithm identifies syndesmophytes in each IDS unit. The cutting algorithm marks as syndesmophyte bone voxels lying between the 2 end plates that bound each IDS. Because of the high precision required by our application, we found it necessary to operate this cutting with subvoxel accuracy [8]. Finally, a last step refines the segmentation of the syndesmophytes using the Laplacian filter and gray level density. The output of the Laplacian filter allowed us to pinpoint the boundary between bone and soft tissue. The interface between the 2 materials can be modeled as a smooth step function. Its Laplacian is positive on one side of the step and negative on the other. Density derived from gray level value allows us to take partial volume effect into account. At the boundary between bone and soft tissue, we added mixed voxels assigning them volumes proportional to their computed bone content [8].

3 Accuracy and Precision of the Algorithm

In a previous study [8], we evaluated the agreement between manually and automatically segmented syndesmophytes using the overlap similarity index (OSI), also known as the Dice similarity coefficient:

$$OSI = \frac{2\,(V_1 \cap V_2)}{V_1 + V_2} \tag{3}$$

where V_1 and V_2 are the two volumes compared. OSI is always comprised between 0 and 1, with 1 indicating perfect overlap. For a random selection of 6 patients, the mean $(+/-$ std) OSI was 0.76 $(+/-$ 0.06).

The precision of the algorithm was evaluated by comparing the results of 2 scans performed on the same day in 9 patients. The protocol was approved by the institutional review board and all subjects provided written informed consent. After the first scan, patients stood up before lying down again for the second scan. This ensured that they did not lie in exactly the same position and that the variation was in the range expected for patients in a longitudinal study. That enabled us to include the variability originating from CT artifacts such as beam hardening. Each patient was scanned from the middle of the T10 vertebra to the middle of the L4 vertebra providing 4 IDSs for analysis. Syndesmophyte volumes from the 4 IDSs were added to form a total per patient. The mean $(+/-$ std) error, 18.3 $(+/-$ 19.6) mm^3, only represents 1.31 % of the total mean syndesmophyte volume, 1,396 $(+/-$ 1,564) mm^3 [17].

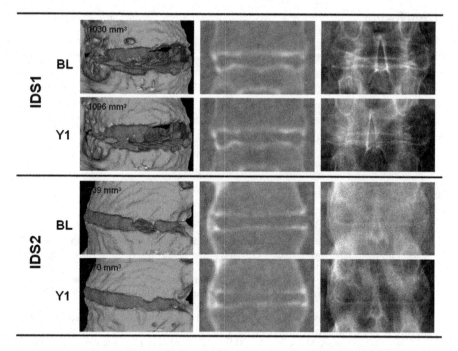

Fig. 4 Two examples of syndesmophyte progression from 2 patients. From *left* to *right*: 3D surface mesh (syndesmophytes in *red* and vertebral bodies in *green*), CT slice, radiograph.

Table 1 Change in syndesmophyte volume (CT) and mSASSS (radiography)

	Mean (+/− std) at baseline	Number of patients with change >0	Mean (+/− std) change
CT	1070 (+/− 1,395) mm³	15 (75%)	92.7 (+/− 196) mm³
Radiography	4.3 (+/− 6.3)	3 (15%)	0.3 (+/− 0.73)

4 Results of the Longitudinal Study

For this study, we performed lumbar spine CT scans on 20 patients at baseline and one year later. The same 4 IDSs as in the precision study were processed. Radiographs of these 4 IDSs were also scored by a physician using the modified Stoke AS Spine Score (mSASSS) [5]. Results from the 4 IDSs were added. Figure 4 shows two examples of syndesmophyte progression detected by the algorithm but not visible on radiographs.

The mean (+/− std) computed syndesmophyte volume change was 92.7 (+/− 196) mm³. 15 patients (75%) had a volume increase while only 3 (15%) had a mSASSS increase (Table 1).

5 Conclusion

To improve the low sensitivity to change associated radiographic reading, we have designed a quantitative measurement of syndesmophytes in CT scans. The method has very good reliability. In a 1 year longitudinal study, the algorithm could detect syndesmophyte growth in 75 % of the patients compared to only 15 % for radiographic reading. This method holds promise for longitudinal clinical studies that need to track syndesmophyte growth.

References

1. Braun, J., Sieper, J.: Ankylosing spondylitis. Lancet **369**, 1379–90 (2007)
2. van der Heijde, D., Landewé, R., Baraliakos, X., et al.: Radiographic findings following two years of infliximab therapy in patients with ankylosing spondylitis. Arthritis Rheum **58**, 3063–3070 (2008)
3. Appel, H., Ruiz-Heiland, G., Listing, J., et al.: Altered skeletal expression of sclerostin and its link to radiographic progression in ankylosing spondylitis. Arthritis Rheum **60**, 3257–3262 (2009)
4. Daoussis, D., Liossis, S.N., Solomou, E.E., et al.: Evidence that Dkk-1 is dysfunctional in ankylosing spondylitis. Arthritis Rheum **62**, 150–158 (2010)
5. Creemers MC, Franssen MJ, van't Hof MA, et al. Assessment of outcome in ankylosing spondylitis: an extended radiographic scoring system. Ann. Rheum. Dis. 64, 127–129 (2005)
6. Spoorenberg, A., de Vlam, K., van der Linden, S., et al.: Radiological scoring methods in ankylosing spondylitis. Reliability and change over 1 and 2 years. J Rheumatol **31**, 125–132 (2004)
7. Tan, S., Yao, J., Ward, M.M., et al.: Computer aided evaluation of ankylosing spondylitis using high-resolution CT. IEEE Trans Med Imaging **27**, 1252–1267 (2008)
8. Tan, S., Yao, J., Yao, L., et al.: Improved precision of syndesmophyte measurement for the evaluation of ankylosing spondylitis using CT: a phantom and patient study. Phys Med Biol **57**, 4683–4704 (2012)
9. Mastmeyer, A., Engelke, K., Fuchs, C., Kalender, W.A.: A hierarchical 3D segmentation method and the definition of vertebral body coordinate systems for QCT of the lumbar spine. Med Image Anal **10**, 560–577 (2006)
10. J. Yao, S.D. O'Connor, R.M. Summers, Automated spinal column extraction and partitioning. In: Proceedings of the IEEE International Symposium on Biomedical Imaging, 390–393 (2006)
11. Aslan, M.S., Ali, A., Rara, H., Farag, A.A.: An automated vertebra identification and segmentation in CT images. In: Proceedings of the IEEE International Conference on Image Processing, 233–236 (2010)
12. Sethian, J.A.: Level set methods and fast marching methods: evolving interfaces in computational geometry, fluid mechanics, computer vision and materials science. Cambridge University Press, Cambridge (1999)
13. Caselles, V., Kimmel, R., Sapiro, G.: Geodesic active contours. Int J Comput Vis **22**, 61–79 (1997)
14. Koenderink J J 1990 Solid Shape: The MIT Press
15. Besl, P.J., McKay, N.D.: A method for registration of 3D shapes. IEEE Trans Pattern Anal Mach Intell **14**, 56–239 (1992)
16. Tan, S., Yao, J., Yao, L.: Summers R M and Ward M M Vertebral surface registration using ridgelines/crestlines Proceedings of SPIEMedical. Imaging **6914**, 69140H (2008)
17. Tan, S., Yao, J., Flynn, J.A., et al.: Quantitative measurement of syndesmophyte volume and height in ankylosing spondylitis using CT. Ann Rheum Dis **73**, 544–550 (2014)

A Semi-automatic Method
for the Quantification of Spinal
Cord Atrophy

**Simon Pezold, Michael Amann, Katrin Weier, Ketut Fundana,
Ernst W. Radue, Till Sprenger and Philippe C. Cattin**

Abstract Due to its high flexibility, the spinal cord is a particularly challenging part
of the central nervous system for the quantification of nervous tissue changes. In this
paper, a novel semi-automatic method is presented that reconstructs the cord surface
from MR images and reformats it to slices that lie perpendicular to its centerline.
In this way, meaningful comparisons of cord cross-sectional areas are possible. Furthermore, the method enables to quantify the complete upper cervical cord volume.
Our approach combines graph cut for presegmentation, edge detection in intensity
profiles for segmentation refinement, and the application of starbursts for reformatting the cord surface. Only a minimum amount of user input and interaction time is
required. To quantify the limits and to demonstrate the robustness of our approach,
its accuracy is validated in a phantom study and its precision is shown in a volunteer
scan–rescan study. The method's reproducibility is compared to similar published
quantification approaches. The application to clinical patient data is presented by
comparing the cord cross-sections of a group of multiple sclerosis patients with
those of a matched control group, and by correlating the upper cervical cord volumes of a large MS patient cohort with the patients' disability status. Finally, we
demonstrate that the geometric distortion correction of the MR scanner is crucial
when quantitatively evaluating spinal cord atrophy.

1 Introduction

Multiple sclerosis (MS) is a chronic inflammatory disorder of the central nervous system that causes both motor disability and cognitive impairment. So far, the diagnosis
and disease monitoring has been based on characteristic patterns of lesions in the
central nervous system that evolve during the disease progression. In recent years,
however, it has been shown that neurodegenerative processes play a central role in

S. Pezold (✉) · M. Amann · K. Weier · K. Fundana · E. W. Radue · T. Sprenger · P. C. Cattin
University Hospital Basel, Basel, Switzerland
e-mail: simon.pezold@unibas.ch

J. Yao et al. (eds.), *Computational Methods and Clinical Applications
for Spine Imaging*, Lecture Notes in Computational Vision and Biomechanics 17,
DOI: 10.1007/978-3-319-07269-2_13, © Springer International Publishing Switzerland 2014

and may be a key to the development of disability [10]. A hallmark of neurodegeneration is atrophy; that is, the loss of nervous tissue. Atrophy can be investigated on a macroscopic scale by using magnetic resonance imaging (MRI), and it has been shown to correlate better with clinical disability than lesion patterns [10]. More specifically, spinal cord (SC) atrophy has been suggested as a biomarker for disease progression, due to the critical role of the SC in motor control [8].

During the last decade, several approaches have been proposed and applied to measure SC cross-sectional areas (CSAs) and volume (e.g., see Miller et al. [9] and Bakshi et al. [2] for methodological overviews), including manual tracing of the SC border as well as semi-automated, intensity-based tracing and subsequent measurement of the resulting CSAs. Common to all these approaches, however, is their requirement for significant user input. A higher degree of automation is therefore desirable to reduce the amount of user input and, with it, the amount of time needed for the usually tedious tasks of manual measurements. More recently, two approaches have been introduced that automatically reconstruct the surface of a manually selected SC section and then successively straighten the result by reformatting it with respect to the SC centerline [4, 6]. In this way, they make it possible to simultaneously assess SC volume changes in a larger region compared to previous approaches.

In this publication, we present a semi-automatic technique that reconstructs the cervical section of the SC surface and then either reformats it to slices perpendicular to the SC centerline or measures the volume of a perpendicularly clipped SC segment. Our method requires only little user input: two small sets of labeled voxels marking both the SC and the background, and one user-provided anatomical landmark to indicate a starting point for the reformatting process. We evaluate the accuracy of our method via a phantom structure of known dimensions. Furthermore, its precision is assessed by analyzing scan–rescan datasets of healthy volunteers. Finally, the applicability to clinical data is shown by comparing the mean CSA of a group of MS patients with an age-matched group of healthy subjects and by referring to a study where our method was successfully applied to correlate upper cervical cord volume with MS disability status. In contrast to the above mentioned methods [4, 6], we put a special focus on how MRI-specific image distortions influence measurements by showing that a distortion correction routine may improve the reproducibility of measurements.

2 Materials

To assess the accuracy of our method, a cylindric perspex phantom filled with copper sulfate–doped water was scanned on a 1.5T whole-body MR scanner (Avanto, Siemens Medical, Germany) with a T1-weighted MPRAGE sequence (TR/TI/TE/α = 2.1 s/1.1 s/3.1 ms/15°); 192 slices in sagittal orientation were acquired with an in-slice resolution of 0.98 mm $\times$ 0.98 mm and a slice thickness of 1 mm. The phantom was scanned in 11 different z-positions relative to the magnetic field center (−50 to 50 mm in increments of 10 mm). The manufacturer's three-dimensional distortion correction routine was applied to the data to see the effects of image distortions induced by gradient non-linearity [7]. Both original and corrected datasets were reconstructed.

To assess the scan–rescan reliability, 12 healthy volunteers (3 female, 9 male, mean age 32.4 y, range 26–44 y) were scanned on a 3T whole-body MR scanner (Verio, Siemens Medical, Germany) with a T1-weighted MPRAGE sequence (TR/TI/TE/α = 2.0 s/1.0 s/3.4 ms/8°); 192 slices in sagittal orientation parallel to the interhemispheric fissure were acquired with an isotropic resolution of 1 mm^3. Both original and distortion-corrected datasets were reconstructed.

To show the applicability to clinical data, 12 relapsing-remitting MS patients (8 female, 4 male, mean age 32.2 y, range 21–46 y; mean disease duration 8.2 y, range 1–17 y, median EDSS 3.0, range 1–4) and 12 age-matched controls (6 female, 6 male, mean age 31.6 y, range 22–48 y) were scanned on a 3T whole-body MR scanner (Verio, Siemens Medical, Germany) with a T1-weighted MPRAGE sequence (TR/TI/TE/α = 1.6 s/0.9 s/2.7 ms/9°); 192 slices in sagittal orientation parallel to the interhemispheric fissure were acquired with an isotropic resolution of 1 mm^3. Distortion-corrected datasets were reconstructed.

3 Method

The proposed method can be broken down into four distinct steps, which we refer to as *presegmentation, segmentation refinement, surface reconstruction,* and *reformatting*. Of these steps, only presegmentation and reformatting need manual intervention while the others run in a completely automated manner. In this way, the user interaction time lies in the order of two to five minutes per scan.

3.1 Presegmentation

The aim of the presegmentation step (see Fig. 1b) is to gain a binary voxel mask that roughly separates the SC section of interest from the background; that is, from the surrounding cerebrospinal fluid (CSF) and all non-cord tissue. While in principle any kind of thresholding technique could be applied, we use graph cuts [3] because of their flexibility and speed. To compensate for intensity differences caused by field inhomogeneities, we apply a bias field correction [11] to the image volumes beforehand. Furthermore, we normalize the image intensities to the [0, 1] interval. We then build a six-connected graph from the voxels around the region of interest (which the user may sketch in transverse, sagittal, and coronal projections of the image volume).

The t-link weights are calculated based on a naive Bayes classifier via the intensity distributions of a set of foreground and background seed points; that is, a selection of voxels labeled by the user as definitely belonging either to the SC or its surroundings.

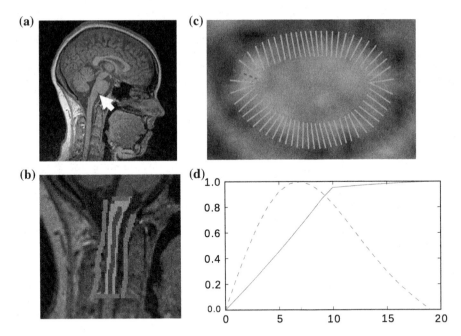

Fig. 1 **a** Location of the *cisterna pontis*. **b** Presegmentation (*blue* region of interest, *red* background seeds, *green* cord seeds, *yellow* result). **c+d** Refinement: **c** intensity profile locations, **d** single intensity profile (*solid*) with smooth derivative estimate (*dashed*), both normalized for display

We model the foreground as a univariate normal distribution and the background as a mixture of four Gaussians. More specifically, we calculate the weights $w_{fg}(x)$ and $w_{bg}(x)$ for the t-links that connect voxel x to the foreground and background terminal, respectively, as

$$
w_{fg}(x) = \begin{cases} \infty & \text{if } x \in \mathscr{F} \\ 0 & \text{if } x \in \mathscr{B} \\ 1 - w_{bg}(x) & \text{else} \end{cases} \quad \text{and} \quad w_{bg}(x) = \begin{cases} 0 & \text{if } x \in \mathscr{F} \\ \infty & \text{if } x \in \mathscr{B} \\ \frac{p_{bg}(I(x))}{p_{bg}(I(x)) + p_{fg}(I(x))} & \text{else} \end{cases},
$$

where $\mathscr{F}$ and $\mathscr{B}$ are the sets of foreground and background seed points, $I(x)$ is the intensity of voxel x, and p_{fg} and p_{bg} are the probability density functions that we estimated from the foreground and background seed point intensities.

The n-link weights $w(x_a, x_b)$ between neighboring voxels x_a and x_b are calculated as $w(x_a, x_b) = \kappa \exp(-0.5\varsigma^{-2}(I(x_a) - I(x_b))^2)$, where $I(x_a)$ and $I(x_b)$ are the respective voxel intensities, κ is a weighting factor, and ς determines the spread of the Gaussian-shaped function (with smaller values for ς leading to a faster decrease of $w(x_a, x_b)$ for increasing differences $I(x_a) - I(x_b)$). The presegmentation is concluded by connected-component labeling, assuring that only the region that includes foreground seeds is retained.

3.2 Segmentation Refinement

Let $I:\Omega \rightarrow \mathbb{R}$ denote the preprocessed (i.e., bias field corrected) image, and let $\mathbf{x} = (x_1, x_2, x_3)^\mathsf{T} \in \Omega$ denote the voxel indices in the image domain $\Omega \subset \mathbb{N}^3$. Furthermore, let $M \subset \Omega$ denote the set of foreground mask voxel indices from the pre-segmentation step. To reduce noise in I, we apply the `GradientAnisotropic-DiffusionImageFilter` of ITK[1] with the conductance parameter fixed to 3.0, the time step fixed to 0.05, and the number of iterations fixed to 20 and 5 for the image used in the first and second pass, respectively. In this way, we yield the denoised images $\hat{I}_1(\mathbf{x})$ and $\hat{I}_2(\mathbf{x})$.

In the first pass, for each transversal slice, we determine the mask boundary voxel indices B_z as

$$B_z = M_z \backslash (M_z \ominus S_4), \tag{1}$$

where $\ominus$ denotes the morphological erosion operator, S_4 is the two-dimensional structuring element representing four-connectivity, and $M_z = \{(x_1, x_2, x_3)^\mathsf{T} \in M : x_3 = z\}$ is the subset of mask voxels for the z-th transversal slice.

We then fit a periodic smoothing B-spline [5] $\mathbf{s}_z(\tau)$ of degree three through the ordered voxel indices $\mathbf{b}_i^z \in B_z$. We distribute the spline's knots $t_i \in [0, 1]$ ($i = 1, \ldots, |B_z|$) according to

$$t_i = \frac{t_i^*}{t_{|B_z|}^*} \quad \text{with} \quad t_1^* = 0 \quad \text{and} \quad t_i^* = t_{i-1}^* + \|\mathbf{b}_i^z - \mathbf{b}_{i-1}^z\|, \tag{2}$$

and constrain the spline smoothness by a smoothing parameter s via

$$\|\mathbf{b}_i^z - \mathbf{s}_z(t_i)\|^2 \le s. \tag{3}$$

The order of the boundary voxels $\mathbf{b}_i^z$ is determined by calculating an estimate of their centroid as $\hat{\mathbf{c}}_z = \frac{1}{|B_z|} \sum_i \mathbf{b}_i^z$ and then sorting them according to the angles formed by the x_1-axis and the vectors $\mathbf{b}_i^z - \hat{\mathbf{c}}_z$. Once we have $\mathbf{s}_z(\tau)$, we divide it into n_1 sections of equal arc length, yielding n_1 new vertices $\mathbf{u}_j^z \in \mathbf{s}_z(\tau)$ ($j = 1, \ldots, n_1$) at the section endpoints. For each $\mathbf{u}_j^z$, we then extract a one-dimensional intensity profile (see Fig. 1c+d) $P_j^z(x)$ with $x \in [0 \ldots k_1 - 1]$ as

$$P_j^z(x) = \hat{I}_1\left(\mathbf{v}_j^z + \delta(x)\right) \quad \text{with} \quad \delta(x) = d_1 \cdot \left(x - \frac{k_1-1}{2}\right)\mathbf{n}_j^z \quad \text{and} \quad \mathbf{v}_j^z = \mathbf{u}_j^z - o\mathbf{n}_j^z, \tag{4}$$

where $\mathbf{n}_j^z$ denotes the unit normal vector pointing inside the spline curve at $\mathbf{u}_j^z$, the resampling distance is given via $d_1 \in \mathbb{R}$, the number of profile samples via $k_1 \in \mathbb{N}$, and $o \in \mathbb{R}$ is an offset to control the profile centering with respect to $\mathbf{u}_j^z$, yielding offset-corrected vertices $\mathbf{v}_j^z$. As our approach to calculate B_z systematically underestimates the mask boundary by half a voxel, we set $o = 0.5$. To get the

---

[1] http://www.itk.org/.

intensity values at the resampling positions x, we use bilinear interpolation in the zth transversal slice of $\hat{I}_1$.

Given that the extracted profiles point to the inside of the spline curve and knowing that in T1-weighted images the inside (i.e., the SC tissue) typically appears brighter than its immediate surroundings (i.e., the CSF), we try to refine the $\mathbf{v}_j^z$ by means of edge detection in the profiles P_j^z. We thus calculate their derivatives as $P_j^{z\prime}(x) = G'(\sigma) * P_j^z(x)$, where $G'(\sigma)$ is the spatial derivative of a Gaussian kernel with standard deviation σ and zero mean. We then search for all local maxima $x_{m,j}$ in $P_j^{z\prime}$ and calculate the new boundary estimate $\mathbf{w}_j^z$ as

$$\mathbf{w}_j^z = \mathbf{v}_j^z + \delta(\hat{x}_{m,j}) \quad \text{with} \quad \hat{x}_{m,j} = \arg\min_{x_{m,j}} \|\delta(x_{m,j})\|. \tag{5}$$

To be less susceptible to noise, we dismiss all $x_{m,j}$ with $P_j^{z\prime}(x_{m,j}) < c \cdot P_j^{z\prime}(x_{\max,j})$ beforehand, where $c \in [0, 1]$ serves as a threshold and $x_{\max,j}$ is the global maximum position of $P_j^{z\prime}$. If no valid maxima are retained, which may be the case if the global maximum value is negative, we set $\mathbf{w}_j^z = \mathbf{v}_j^z$.

A second pass of boundary estimation follows, similar to the first pass, starting with the $\mathbf{w}_j^z$ as initial estimate. The only differences are the following: first, to ensure a homogeneous distribution of the boundary estimates, particularly with regard to the surface reconstruction step (Sect. 3.3), the fitted spline is now resampled n_2 times at equal *angular* distances, using the spline center as point of reference, yielding redistributed estimates $\mathbf{y}_j^z$ ($j = 1, \ldots, n_2$). Second, the new intensity profiles $Q_j^z(x)$ with $x \in [0...k_2 - 1]$ are extracted as

$$Q_j^z(x) = \hat{I}_2\left(\mathbf{y}_j^z + d_2 \cdot \left(x - \frac{k_2-1}{2}\right) \frac{\nabla \hat{I}_2^z(y_1, y_2)}{\|\nabla \hat{I}_2^z(y_1, y_2)\|}\right) \quad \text{with} \quad (y_1, y_2, z)^\mathsf{T} = \mathbf{y}_j^z; \tag{6}$$

that is, no offset is added and the normalized gradient vectors of the in-slice intensities $\hat{I}_2^z$ at $\mathbf{y}_j^z$ replace the spline normal vector. The boundary re-estimation is calculated analogous to Eq. (5), leading to the final boundary position $\mathbf{z}_j^z$.

As a result of the refinement procedure, we now have n_2 vertices $\mathbf{z}_j^z$ for all of those transversal slices that contain foreground mask voxels. These vertices represent the slice-wise SC contour at subvoxel precision, provided that the profile resampling distances d_1 and d_2 were chosen sufficiently small.

3.3 Surface Reconstruction

We transform the $\mathbf{z}_j^z$ to their locations $\mathbf{a}_j^z$ in the metric world coordinate system by means of a transformation matrix determined from the image source's meta data. We then connect each $\mathbf{a}_j^z$ to $\mathbf{a}_j^{z+1}$, $\mathbf{a}_{j+1}^z$, and $\mathbf{a}_{j+1}^{z+1}$, which results in strips of $2n_2$

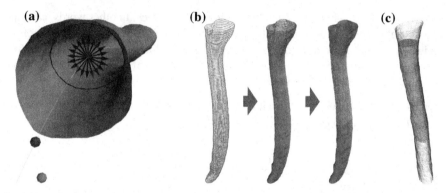

Fig. 2 a Reformatting (*yellow* centerline, *green* landmark and anchor point, *blue* simplified star-burst and new contour). **b** Schematic reformatting steps: contour stacking, surface reconstruction, reslicing. **c** Perpendicular volume clipping (*gray* original surface, *blue* clipped volume segment)

triangles between each pair of successive slices and thus in a complete SC surface reconstruction S for the initially masked region of interest (see Fig. 2b).

3.4 Reformatting

To compare different image volumes, spatial correspondence has to be established between them. In our setting we have to make sure that anatomically corresponding SC locations are compared. This is not straightforward for two reasons: first, the SC can be bent rather differently in the head and neck area between scans; and second, the SC slides along the spinal canal during this bending, making landmarks such as the vertebrae or intervertebral discs unsuitable.

We identified the *cisterna pontis*, a distinct indentation at the caudal *pons*, as a landmark that may easily be spotted and manually marked (see Fig. 1a). Moreover, the landmark is a structure that is part of the nervous tissue and, as such, stays in a fixed position relative to the SC. This may be a benefit compared to other features located on the intervertebral discs [6, 8] or on bone structures such as the *foramen magnum* [4], which are more likely to be susceptible to relocation due to bending. To the best of our knowledge, the *cisterna pontis* has not been described as a landmark in the context of SC surface reconstructions.

Concerning the bending, we propose a similar approach as previously described by Coulon et al. [4]. Let $\mathbf{c}_z$ describe the centroid of the polygon formed by the vertices $\mathbf{a}_j^z$; let $z = 1, \ldots, m$ here serve as an index variable that consecutively numbers all m transversal slices containing parts of the surface reconstruction S. We then define the centerline $\mathbf{c}(\tau)$ of S as a smoothing B-spline of degree three through the $\mathbf{c}_z$ (Sect. 3.2). Let $\mathbf{p} \in \mathbb{R}^3$ denote the position of the *cisterna pontis* landmark in world coordinates. The anchor point $\mathbf{c}_0 = \mathbf{c}(\tau_0)$ for reformatting is then determined by the condition

$(\mathbf{p} - \mathbf{c}_0) \cdot \mathbf{c}_0' = 0$, where $\mathbf{c}_0'$ is a spline tangent vector in $\mathbf{c}_0$; in other words, $\mathbf{c}_0$ is an orthogonal projection of $\mathbf{p}$ onto the spline curve. We extrapolate the superior spline end if necessary to find a τ_0 and $\mathbf{c}_0$ that satisfy the condition. Depending on whether one intends to measure reformatted CSAs or the volume of a SC section, either the reslicing steps or the volume measurement steps described below follow.

Reslicing. For measuring reformatted CSAs, a total of n_3 reslicing positions $\mathbf{c}_i = \mathbf{c}(\tau_i)$ $(i = 1, \ldots, n_3)$ are determined by solving

$$\int_{\tau_0}^{\tau_i} \left\| \frac{d\mathbf{c}}{d\tau} \right\| d\tau = \omega + (i - 1)d_3 \tag{7}$$

with respect to τ_i; in other words, the $\mathbf{c}_i$ are calculated at intervals of equal arc length d_3 along the spline curve, starting from $\mathbf{c}_0$, with an offset ω.

Based on the $\mathbf{c}_i$, we want to reformat the surface reconstruction S to slices that lie perpendicular to the centerline $\mathbf{c}$. Formally speaking, we thus require for each $\mathbf{c}_i$ the set of surface points $C_i \subset S$ that satisfy $C_i = R_i \cap S$ with $R_i = \{\mathbf{r}: (\mathbf{r} - \mathbf{c}_i) \cdot \mathbf{c}_i' = 0\}$; that is, we require the points that lie in the intersections of S with the planes $R_i \perp \mathbf{c}$ through the reslicing positions $\mathbf{c}_i$.

In practice, we calculate approximations of these intersections. For this, we build n_3 bundles of rays, hereafter referred to as 'starbursts'. Each starburst (see Fig. 2a) consists of n_4 rays $\mathbf{q}_j^i$ $(j = 1, \ldots, n_4)$ given by

$$\mathbf{q}_j^i(\lambda) = \mathbf{c}_i + \lambda \mathbf{r}_j^i \quad \text{with} \quad \lambda \geq 0, \quad \|\mathbf{r}_j^i\| = 1, \quad \text{and} \quad \mathbf{r}_j^i \cdot \mathbf{c}_i' = 0. \tag{8}$$

The direction vectors $\mathbf{r}_j^i$ are directed at equal angular intervals around $\mathbf{c}_i$; that is, $\forall j : \mathbf{r}_j^i \cdot \mathbf{r}_{j+1}^i = \cos(\frac{2\pi}{n_4})$. The actual reslicing procedure amounts to a series of ray–triangle intersections of all $\mathbf{q}_j^i$ with the triangles that form S. As a result, we get a new set of $n_3 \cdot n_4$ vertices $\mathbf{b}_j^i \in C_i$, which for each of the n_3 positions may be connected to a polygon serving as a contour representation for the respective reformatted slice. These contours are finally suitable for CSA measurements that make inter-scan comparisons possible.

Volume Measurement. For measuring the volume of an SC section of length l, the surface reconstruction S is clipped by two planes that are located at arc lengths ω and $\omega + l$ measured along the centerline (see Eq. 7) and that lie perpendicular to the respective centerline tangent vectors. We then close the ends of the clipped section and calculate the volume of the resulting closed surface (see Fig. 2c) based on the divergence theorem [1].

4 Results

To assess the performance of our proposed algorithm, we conducted experiments on phantom, scan–rescan, and real patient data. For all these experiments, the following parameter settings were applied: $\kappa = 0.4$, $\varsigma = 0.5$, $s = 3.0$ voxels (splines in the refinement step), $s = 3.5$ mm (centerline splines), $n_{1,2,4} = 60$, $k_{1,2} = 20$, $d_1 = 0.2$ voxels, $d_2 = 0.1$ voxels, $c = 0.3$, $\sigma = 0.5$ voxels, $d_3 = 0.25$ mm. If not stated differently, reslicing took place in superior–inferior direction over a length of 50 mm, resulting in $n_3 = 201$ new slices.

Phantom Evaluation. Among other structures, the used phantom contains a solid cylindric structure, surrounded by a liquid-filled cavity, of 60 mm length and 25 mm diameter (corresponding to a CSA of 490.9 mm^2), which was roughly aligned with the scanner's z-axis during the scans. As a substitute for the SC landmark, we placed a marker at the most posterior point of the structure's boundary in the most superior slice where its CSA was still completely visible and set $\omega = 2$ mm.

In the uncorrected scans, the mean CSA was 504.7 ± 1.8 mm^2, thus the true CSA was overestimated by approximately 2.8 %. In the corrected scans, the mean CSA was 503.0 ± 1.3 mm^2, thus the true CSA was overestimated by approximately 2.5 %.

Scan–Rescan Evaluation. For the scan–rescan evaluation, the twelve subjects were scanned three times in a row (scans S1, S2, S3). Between S1 and S2 they were asked not to move so that the SC location and bending would be as similar as possible in both scans. Between S2 and S3 the subjects had to exit the scanner and were repositioned afterwards. One subject was excluded because the *cisterna pontis* was not visible in all scans. To measure the intra-observer reproducibility, the distortion-corrected S1 scans were presegmented twice by one observer, with a period of more than one month between associated presegmentations. To measure the inter-observer reproducibility, the distortion-corrected S1 scans were presegmented independently by a second observer.

We focused on two different aspects for interpreting the results: the effects of the distortion correction routine, and the comparison to published SC segmentation methods.

In a first experiment (E1), we set the reslicing offset to $\omega = 50$ mm and measured the CSAs in superior–inferior direction over a length of 15 mm (resulting in 61 new slices), approximately covering the caudal end of the C2 vertebra. We then averaged the CSA for the reformatted contours of each scan and calculated the coefficient of variation (CV; i.e., the sample standard deviation over the mean) for comparisons of S1 and S2, S1 and S3 (both in the corrected and the uncorrected scans), as well as for the intra-observer and inter-observer comparisons. This setup was chosen in order to compare our results with the method described by Losseff et al. [8], who measure the average CSA of the caudal C2 end over five slices of 3 mm thickness that were reformatted to lie perpendicular to the SC orientation.

In a second experiment (E2), in order to compare our results with the methods described by Coulon et al. [4] and Horsfield et al. [6], we set the reslicing offset

Table 1 Coefficients of variation, distortion-corrected versus uncorrected scans (%)

	E1: C2 Avg. CSA		E2: C1–C3 Avg. CSA		E2: C1–C3 Volume		E3: C1–C3 Slice-wise CSA	
	S1–S2	S1–S3	S1–S2	S1–S3	S1–S2	S1–S3	S1–S2	S1–S3
Uncorrected	0.42	1.55	0.36	1.90	0.35	1.89	1.16	2.48
Corrected	0.42	**1.15**	**0.33**	**0.94**	**0.33**	**0.93**	**1.10**	**1.76**

to $\omega = 25$ mm and segmented over our default length of 50 mm. In this way, we covered a wider region of the cervical SC, namely approximately the section between the cranial end of the C1 and the caudal end of the C3 vertebra. For each scan, we then calculated the mean CSA over the reformatted contours of the complete region as well as the region's perpendicularly clipped volume. The CVs were calculated for the same combinations as described in the first experiment.

In a third experiment (E3), we wanted to see whether our method is applicable to not only measure a mean CSA, but also to measure the CSA on specific levels along the SC reliably. We thus swapped the order of averaging and CV calculation: first, we calculated a CV for the contours on the same level (e.g., the CV for the first reformatted contour in the S1–S2 comparison for subject one), then we averaged over the CVs for each comparison.

Effects of the distortion correction routine. A comparison of the mean CVs over all subjects for the distortion-corrected and uncorrected scans is shown in Table 1. The results conform to our expectations. As the S1–S2 position change was minimal, the image distortions have little influence here. This is because they affect both scan and rescan similarly, and thus the S1–S2 CVs are on the same level for the corrected and uncorrected scans. After repositioning (i.e., S1–S3), however, the uncorrected data CVs become distinctly worse than the corrected data CVs, showing the benefit of the correction routine as soon as scan conditions are not perfectly similar anymore. Furthermore, the S1–S3 corrected data CVs are also worse than their S1–S2 equivalents, which suggests that the correction routine does not account for all geometric distortions in the scans. Partial volume effects, for example, may be another contributor to variations in the reconstructions and thus in the subsequent measurements.

Comparison with published methods. For all experiments, the mean CVs over all subjects are reported in Table 2, making use of the distortion-corrected scans for our method. The results of Experiments 1 and 2 compare favorably with the values reported by Losseff et al. [8], Coulon et al. [4], and Horsfield et al. [6]. The low intra- and inter-observer CVs show the strength of our method in that the outcome is very robust given different presegmentation inputs, whether produced by the same observer or different observers.

The results of Experiment 3 indicate that even measurements on single-contour level may produce reasonable outcomes with our method. To put these values into perspective: given a realistic CSA of 75 mm^2, changes of 0.91 mm^2 (1.96 standard deviations) on a specific slice should be detectable in distortion-corrected scans with

Table 2 Coefficients of variation, comparison with published methods (%)

		Scan–rescan		Intra-observer	Inter-observer
		S1–S2	S1–S3		
E1	Our method, C2 average CSA	0.42	1.15	**0.15**	**0.14**
	Horsfield et al. [6], C2 average CSA	–	–	0.59	1.36
	Losseff et al. [8], experienced observer	–	**0.79**	0.73	–
	Losseff et al. [8], inexperienced observer	–	1.61	1.03	–
E2	Our method, C1–C3 average CSA	0.33	**0.94**	**0.28**	**0.36**
	Horsfield et al. [6], C2–C5 average CSA	–	–	0.44	1.07
	Coulon et al. [4], average CSA	–	1.31	0.77	–
	Our method, C1–C3 volume	0.33	**0.93**	**0.26**	0.35
	Coulon et al. [4], volume	–	1.35	1.36	–
E3	Our method, C1–C3 slice-wise CSA	1.10	1.76	0.62	0.70

95 % confidence by the same observer.[2] Assuming a CSA of circular shape, this corresponds to a change in radius of 0.03 mm.

Preliminary Evaluation on Patient Data. One distortion-corrected scan per subject was used for the cross-sectional clinical data evaluation. The SC surfaces were reconstructed and resliced with an offset of $\omega = 25$ mm, and the SC volume was measured over the default 50 mm section. One patient was excluded afterwards because the reconstruction showed substantial spike artefacts in the inferior part caused by some refinement line profiles erroneously capturing the edge of the surrounding vertebra. The mean SC volume was $3{,}464 \pm 592$ mm^3 for the patient group and $3{,}811 \pm 444$ mm^3 for the control group. For both the patient group and the control group, we also calculated the mean slice-wise CSAs. As can be seen in Fig. 3, the patient CSA is smaller than that of the healthy controls throughout all slices. Comparing the mean slice-wise CSAs on each level in a paired-samples t-test showed a statistically significant difference ($p < 0.01$) between the two groups.

Evaluation on a Large MS Patient Cohort. In a recent publication [12], we applied our method to a cohort of 172 MS patients. Perpendicularly clipped SC volumes were measured as described above, with an offset of $\omega = 20$ mm. In a hierarchical multiple linear regression analysis including demographic factors as well as volumetric measures and MS lesion load, the SC volume was shown to be one of the strongest predictors ($p < 0.001$; $\beta = -0.28$) of the Expanded Disability Status Scale (EDSS) score, which signifies the clinically determined degree of disability. In this way, both similar results of other studies were confirmed (such as the ones mentioned in [10]) and the applicability of our method to clinical data was demonstrated.

---

[2] Note that this is *not* the same value as the 0.67 mm^2 reported by Horsfield et al. [6] in a similar argument for the C2–C5 region, as they describe the CV of average CSAs, while we describe an average CV over slice-wise CSAs here. If we do the same calculation for our method with the C1–C3 average CSA (see Table 2, E2), assuming a CSA of 78 mm^2 as reported in [6], the detectable change even drops to 0.43 mm^2.

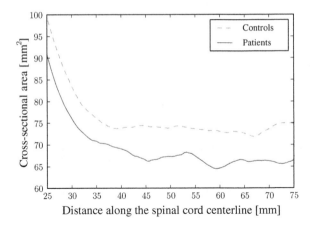

Fig. 3 Mean cross-sectional area along the spinal cord centerline for the MS patient and control group, distances measured relative to the reformatting anchor point

5 Conclusion

We presented a novel semi-automatic method for the reconstruction and reformatting of the spinal cord surface that enables reliable comparisons of both the complete upper cervical cord area and the cord cross-sectional areas over the range of several vertebrae, even if different degrees of spine bending occur between scans. The accuracy of our method was demonstrated by measurements on phantom data. We could also show that a minimum amount of interaction time (two to five minutes) and user-provided input (two sets of labeled voxels and one anatomical landmark) are sufficient to acquire highly reproducible results. These results reach a comparable if not superior precision level with respect to similar approaches [4, 6] (coefficient of variation values <1 % for mean CSAs and volumes, values in the 1–2 % range for slice-wise CSAs). Furthermore, we showed that the application of a correction routine to account for geometric distortions induced by gradient non-linearity increases the degree of reproducibility. The latter appears to us to be an important aspect that nevertheless has been neglected (or has at least not been mentioned explicitly) by similar cord reconstruction approaches (cf. [4, 6]), so far.

Finally, the method's applicability to clinical data was demonstrated by a comparison of the slice-wise cross-sectional areas of a group of MS patients with an age-matched control group. We could later confirm these preliminary results by successfully correlating SC volumes with disability scores in a large cohort of MS patients, thus showing the suitability of our approach for everyday use.

Acknowledgments This work was supported by the MIAC Corporation, University Hospital Basel, Switzerland.

References

1. Alyassin, A.M., Lancaster III, J.L., Downs, J.H., Fox, P.T.: Evaluation of new algorithms for the interactive measurement of surface area and volume. Med. Phys. **21**(6), 741–752 (1994)
2. Bakshi, R., Dandamudi, V.S.R., Neema, M., De, C., Bermel, R.A.: Measurement of brain and spinal cord atrophy by magnetic resonance imaging as a tool to monitor multiple sclerosis. J. Neuroimaging **15**, 30S–45S (2005)
3. Boykov, Y.Y., Jolly, M.P.: Interactive graph cuts for optimal boundary & region segmentation of objects in n-d images. In: Eighth IEEE International Conference on Computer Vision, 2001. ICCV 2001. Proceedings, vol. 1, pp. 105–112 (2001)
4. Coulon, O., Hickman, S.J., Parker, G.J., Barker, G.J., Miller, D.H., Arridge, S.R.: Quantification of spinal cord atrophy from magnetic resonance images via a b-spline active surface model. Mag. Reson. Med. **47**(6), 1176–1185 (2002)
5. Dierckx, P.: Algorithms for smoothing data with periodic and parametric splines. Comput. Graph. Image Process. **20**(2), 171–184 (1982)
6. Horsfield, M.A., Sala, S., Neema, M., Absinta, M., Bakshi, A., Sormani, M.P., Rocca, M.A., Bakshi, R., Filippi, M.: Rapid semi-automatic segmentation of the spinal cord from magnetic resonance images: application in multiple sclerosis. NeuroImage **50**(2), 446–455 (2010)
7. Jovicich, J., Czanner, S., Greve, D., Haley, E., van der Kouwe, A., Gollub, R., Kennedy, D., Schmitt, F., Brown, G., MacFall, J., Fischl, B., Dale, A.: Reliability in multi-site structural MRI studies: effects of gradient non-linearity correction on phantom and human data. NeuroImage **30**(2), 436–443 (2006)
8. Losseff, N.A., Webb, S.L., O'Riordan, J.I., Page, R., Wang, L., Barker, G.J., Tofts, P.S., McDonald, W.I., Miller, D.H., Thompson, A.J.: Spinal cord atrophy and disability in multiple sclerosis. Brain **119**(3), 701–708 (1996)
9. Miller, D.H., Barkhof, F., Frank, J.A., Parker, G.J.M., Thompson, A.J.: Measurement of atrophy in multiple sclerosis: pathological basis, methodological aspects and clinical relevance. Brain **125**(8), 1676–1695 (2002)
10. Reynolds, R., Roncaroli, F., Nicholas, R., Radotra, B., Gveric, D., Howell, O.: The neuropathological basis of clinical progression in multiple sclerosis. Acta Neuropathol. **122**(2), 155–170 (2011)
11. Tustison, N., Avants, B., Cook, P., Zheng, Y., Egan, A., Yushkevich, P., Gee, J.: N4ITK: improved n3 bias correction. IEEE Trans. Med. Imaging **29**(6), 1310–1320 (2010)
12. Weier, K., Pezold, S., Andelova, M., Amann, M., Magon, S., Naegelin, Y., Radue, E.W., Stippich, C., Gass, A., Kappos, L., Cattin, P., Sprenger, T.: Both spinal cord volume and spinal cord lesions impact physical disability in multiple sclerosis. Multiple Sclerosis J. **19**(Suppl), 188–189 (2013)

Part IV
Segmentation II (MR)

Multi-modal Vertebra Segmentation from MR Dixon for Hybrid Whole-Body PET/MR

Christian Buerger, Jochen Peters, Irina Waechter-Stehle,
Frank M. Weber, Tobias Klinder and Steffen Renisch

Abstract In this paper, a novel model-based segmentation of the vertebrae is introduced that uses multi-modal image features from Dixon MR images (i.e. water/fat separated). Our primary application is the segmentation of the bony anatomy for the generation of attenuation maps in hybrid PET/MR imaging systems. The focus of this work is on the geometric accuracy of the segmentation from MR. From ground-truth structure delineations on training data sets, image features for a model-based segmentation are trained on both the water and fat images from the Dixon series. For the actual segmentation, both features are used simultaneously to improve both robustness and accuracy compared to single image segmentations. The method is validated on 25 patients by comparing the results to semi-automatically generated ground truth annotations. A mean surface distance error of 1.69 mm over all vertebrae is achieved, leading to an improvement of up to 41 % compared to using a single image alone.

1 Introduction

Recently emerging hybrid whole-body imaging systems where magnetic resonance (MR) imaging is combined with positron emission tomography (PET) are highly interesting for a variety of clinical indications, e.g. in oncology. While PET provides functional information with high sensitivity, MR (i) provides superior soft tissue contrast for excellent anatomical localization and (ii) can be used to generate maps that correct PET for attenuation.

From an image acquisition point of view, MR Dixon sequences have recently been investigated to generate such attenuation maps. Using Dixon techniques, soft tissue

C. Buerger (✉) · J. Peters · I. Waechter-Stehle · F. M. Weber · T. Klinder · S. Renisch
Department of Digital Imaging, Philips Technologie GmbH, Innovative Technologies, Research
Laboratories, Hamburg, Germany
e-mail: christian.buerger@philips.com

J. Yao et al. (eds.), *Computational Methods and Clinical Applications*
for Spine Imaging, Lecture Notes in Computational Vision and Biomechanics 17,
DOI: 10.1007/978-3-319-07269-2_14, © Springer International Publishing Switzerland 2014

can easily be separated into its water and fat components; with moderate additional effort attenuation maps with four compartments (background, lung tissue, muscle and connective watery tissue, and fatty tissue) can be generated [1]. Cortical bone tissue, such as the vertebrae, does not provide signal in standard MR sequences and commonly ignored during attenuation correction (AC) which can lead to substantial errors especially for metastases located close to bone [2]. Ultrashort echo time (UTE) sequences have been proposed and successfully been combined with Dixon imaging to include bone tissue in AC of the head [3]. However, UTE is still prone to imaging artifacts and long scan times with respect to whole-body applications. Consequently, extracting bone tissue such as the vertebrae from MR Dixon images using image processing would allow accurate AC without the need of time-consuming UTE scans.

Various groups have investigated image processing techniques to segment the vertebrae or intervertebral disks from MR images. Intensity based semi-automatic [4] and automatic [5, 6] approaches have been presented. More advanced techniques that are based on deformable models have been investigated [7, 8] and show potential to be more robust against MR imaging artifacts (caused by medical implants, low spatial resolution, or other image artifacts). All of these approaches, however, use a single MR image for vertebra detection, most commonly a T1- or a T2-weighted MR image. In PET/MR, Dixon MR images can also be used for segmentation. These images are clinically well accepted for anatomical localization and (i) provide additional contrast with intrinsically perfect registration, and (ii) avoid artifacts related to chemical shift. However, image contrast varies between the water and fat image: in some cases the image contrast around the vertebrae is better in the water image (and would be favorable for segmentation), in other cases the contrast is better in the fat image (and would be favorable for segmentation). In other words, a segmentation is desired that takes advantage of both the water and fat contrast. While image compounding methods have been proposed to fuse multiple images into a single image with optimal contrast [9], segmentation from multiple images simultaneously would avoid a potential insertion of compounding artifacts and a potential loss of valuable information.

In this paper, we adapt a 3D model-based segmentation framework described in [10] to automatically extract seventeen vertebrae (from sacrum to neck: lumbar vertebra 1–5 as well as thoracic vertebra 1–12) from a Dixon MR acquisition (note that our focus is on MR-based segmentation while the application to AC of PET is subject to future work). The segmentation approach is based on adapting a single mesh to multiple images, the water and fat image. During adaptation, each point on the mesh surface is attracted by feature points that are once detected in the water image and another time in the fat image. These multi-modal features used within a single segmentation are the main novel contribution of this paper. We present segmentation results from 25 patients and compare our results with segmentations using only the water or the fat image alone. We validate our method using manually corrected semi-automatic ground truth data and achieve a segmentation accuracy (mesh surface distances) of 1.69 mm, an improvement of 41 and 24 % compared to the water and fat segmentation, respectively.

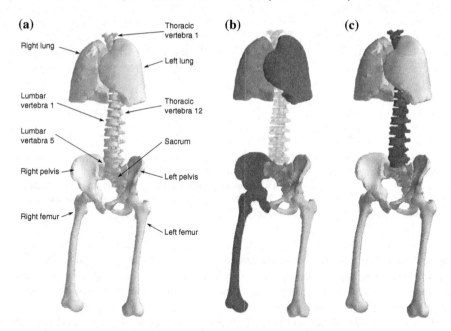

Fig. 1 Segmentation model and segmentation pipeline. **a** The model compartments being used for model localization (based on the generalized Hough transform). **b** Parametric adaptation. Individual affine transformations are assigned to the "anchoring structures" femur/pelvis/lungs. The vertebrae are deactivated in this step (transparent) to avoid wrong mesh to image vertebra assignments. All vertebrae are positioned according to the remaining components. **c** Deformable adaptation. In this final step, the segmentation is refined using local mesh deformations. All vertebrae are consecutively activated and adapted to the image (from sacrum to neck) to ensure correct vertebra labelings

2 Methods

The segmentation framework is based on adapting a surface model represented as a triangulated mesh to a given input image. Section 2.1 describes the segmentation pipeline, and Sect. 2.2 describes our main contribution of incorporating multi-modal image features.

2.1 Segmentation

The surface model being used as shape prior for segmentation is shown in Fig. 1a. Since a direct vertebra segmentation from whole-body images is prone to localization errors, we choose a combined model that includes tissues that serve as "anchoring strucures" for the vertebrae: (1) femur/pelvis and (2) lungs. Note that both femur and pelvis were chosen as anchoring structures in the pelvic region because they showed most reliable segmentation results due to clear image deliniations between bone and

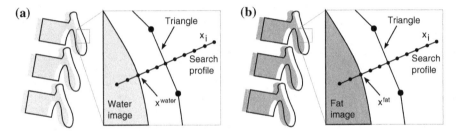

Fig. 2 Target point detection using multi-modal image features. For each mesh triangle, a search profile is defined along the perpendicular triangle direction. Target points x^{water} and x^{fat} are detected as the one points that maximize a feature response (such as the maximum image gradient) in the water (**a**) and in the fat image (**b**), respectively. During adaptation, the mesh triangle is simultaneously attracted to x^{water} as well as to x^{fat}

soft tissue. In other words, we first segment femur/pelvis/lungs to initially place the vertebrae at their approximate position (i.e. within the capture range), before they are locally adapted to the image. The segmentation pipeline consists of three steps (see [10] for details):

Step 1. Model localization. In this first step, the model is located in the image at the approximately correct position. The localizer is based on the generalized Hough Transform (GHT) and attempts to align mesh triangles with image gradients. *Step 2. Parametric adaptation.* Multiple rigid/affine transformations of the anchoring structures (different colors in Fig. 1b) allow registration of these structures with the image. In this step all vertebrae are deactivated (transparent in Fig. 1b) to avoid wrong anatomical correspondences between mesh and image vertebra. They are rather passively scaled and positioned at their approximate location in the image based on the transformations of the anchoring structures. *Step 3. Deformable adaptation.* In this final step, first all anchoring structures are simultaneously adapted to the image using local deformations. The vertebrae are then successively activated (from sacrum to neck) to ensure a correct localization of each individual vertebra: first the lumbar vertebra 5 is activated and adapted to the image, then the next lumbar vertebra 4 is activated and adapted, then lumbar vertebra 3, etc. (Fig. 1c). This iterative activation and adaptation is repeated until the top thoracic vertebra 1 is reached.

2.2 Multi-modal Features

During parametric as well as during deformable adaptation, the mesh triangles are attracted to image target points detected by the following algorithm (Fig. 2). For each mesh triangle, we construct a search profile (perpendicular to the triangle) of $2l$ points x_i with $i \in [-l, l]$ and search for a target point that maximizes an image feature response $F(x_i)$

$$x = \arg\max_{\{x_i\}} [F(x_i)].$$ (1)

Each feature $F(x_i)$ evaluates the image gradient strength and checks the local image appearance such as trained intensity values. For instance, edges may be rejected if the intensity values at the inner and outer side of a triangle do not match the trained expectation. Note that these trained intensity values are modality-specific.

While commonly a single modality, or image, is being used for feature detection, we use multiple modalities (here the Dixon water and fat images). Figure 2 illustrates these multi-modal image features for a single triangle. First, the triangle attempts to detect a target point x^{water} in the water image (Fig. 2a). Second, the same triangle attempts to detect a target point x^{fat} in the fat image (Fig. 2b). This approach is repeated for all triangles on the mesh to derive a sequence of water target points x_t^{water} as well as a sequence of fat target points x_t^{fat}. During adaptation an external energy term is minimized that simultaneously attracts the mesh triangles to all x_t^{water} as well as to all x_t^{fat}. A simplified energy formulation from [10] can be described as:

$$E_{ext} = \sum_{t=0}^{T} \left[c_t - x_t^{water} \right]^2 + \sum_{t=0}^{T} \left[c_t - x_t^{fat} \right]^2,$$ (2)

where c_t is the triangle center with index t, and T is the number of mesh triangles.

To allow target point detections as shown in Fig. 2, image features were trained (see [11] for details) from ground truth annotations which were generated in a bootstrap-like approach. An initial model (with $\sim$1000 triangles forming the mesh surface of a each vertebra) was manually adapted to the images of the first subject. This annotation was used for independent feature training on the water and fat image, respectively. The resulting model was adapted to the images of the second subject (using multi-modal image features as described above) and manually corrected if required. This annotation was included in a new feature training and the resulting model was applied to the images of the next subject. This process was repeated until ground truth annotations from all patients were available.

Example images of a single patient, *Pat1*, and the resulting image features from all trainings are shown in Fig. 3, for the water (Fig. 3a) and for the fat image (Fig. 3b). As can be observed, water and fat features vary for all vertebrae, and one cannot always decide which feature is optimal. Segmenting both the water and the fat image simultaneously is expected to provide more robust and accurate segmentation results compared to using the water or fat features alone.

(a)   **(b)**

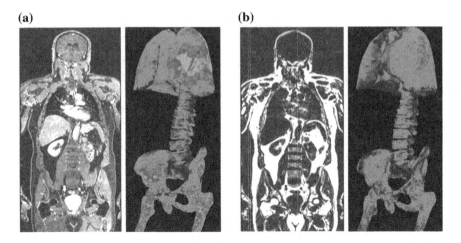

Fig. 3 Trained image features. **a** Water image from a single patient, *Pat1*, and the water feature quality in terms of simulated errors (see [11]) being trained on all patients. **b** Fat image from *Pat1* and the fat feature quality being estimated from all patients. The color scale shows high quality features (*green*) to low quality features (*red*). As can be observed, water features are better around the lungs, femur, and pelvis. However, features around the vertebrae appear similar, and a simultaneous segmentation on both the water and fat image is expected to provide most reliable results

3 Experiments

3.1 Materials

Dixon MR images from 25 patients were acquired on a 3T MR Scanner (Philips Ingenuity TF PET/MR, Best, The Netherlands) using a quadrature body coil, with $TR / TE_1 / TE_2 = 3.2/1.11/2.0$ ms and flip angle $10°$. Seven bed stations were acquired (30 mm overlap) to cover a field of view (FOV) from head to thigh. Each station was acquired with a FOV of $500 \times 400 \times 150$ mm^3 (right-left, anterior-posterior, feet-head), reconstructed axial resolution 0.8×0.8 mm^2, 3 mm slice thickness, scan duration 17 s.

3.2 Segmentation

To separate the training set from the test set, a five fold cross approach was employed. All 25 patients were randomly grouped in five subsets. Four of the five subsets (20 patients) were used for training, the remaining one subset (5 patients) was used for segmentation. Segmentation accuracy was validated using mesh surface distances to the ground truth annotations. For each vertebra, we computed the mean distances over all triangles as well as the amount of triangles with errors of larger than 5 mm.

The proposed multi-modal feature segmentation was also compared with single image segmentations. Three experiments were performed: (i) segmentation of the water image using water features, (ii) segmentation of the fat image using fat features, and (iii) segmentation of both the water and the fat image simultaneously using the proposed multi-modal image features. Note that for all experiments multi-modal features were used for initial model placement (*Step 1* and *Step 2* from Sect. 2.1), and the feature comparison was only performed in the last local adaptation step (*Step 3. Deformable adaptation*).

4 Results

The segmentation steps of our adaptation pipeline using the proposed multi-modal image features are shown in Fig. 4 (overlaid onto both the water and fat image). Figure 4a shows the model initialization, i.e. the initial placement of the mean model according to the GHT. The segmentation is then refined in Fig. 4b using parametric transformations. After this step, all vertebrae are approximately at their correct positions and within the capture range of the deformable adaptation. During the last deformable adaptation (Fig. 4c), all mesh components including the vertebrae are locally adapted to the image which completes the segmentation.

Figure 5 shows results from four other patients, showing vertebra segmentations in sagittal view, again overlaid onto the water and the fat images. As can be observed, our approach successfully segmented the vertebrae in all examples. Compared to the ground truth annotations over all vertebrae, a maximum mean error of 1.81 mm (6.40 % of the triangles showing an error of >5 mm) was observed for *Pat4*. Figure 6 shows a segmentation comparison when (i) using only water features, (ii) using only fat features and (iii) using the proposed multi-modal (water and fat) features for two other patiens, *Pat7* and *Pat8*. For *Pat7*, segmentation using water features only showed large errors of up 14.27 mm (thoracic vertebra 4, arrow in Fig. 6a). Image contrast appears low in that region and the water model was not able to provide accurate segmentation. Similarly, for *Pat8*, the segmentation using fat features only showed large errors of up to 15.48 mm (thoracic vertebra 6, arrow in Fig. 6b). For comparison, segmentation using multi-modal image features (Fig. 6c) provided accurate results for both patients with maximum errors of 4.00 mm (thoracic vertebra 5) and 4.75 mm (thoracic vertebra 7), respectively.

Table 1 shows results for each vertebra in the mean over all 25 patients, from lumbar vertebra 5 (close to pelvis) to thoracic vertebra 1 (close to neck). Considering all vertebrae and all patients, using the water and fat images alone led to a segmentation error of 2.89 mm (15.90 % with >5 mm error) and 2.22 mm (9.43 %), respectively. Our proposed multi-modal feature approach showed a clear reduction to 1.69 mm (5.17 %). Note that for all feature cases, the top thoracic vertebra 1 showed the largest error due to low image constrast in most images.

(a)   Water image   Fat image

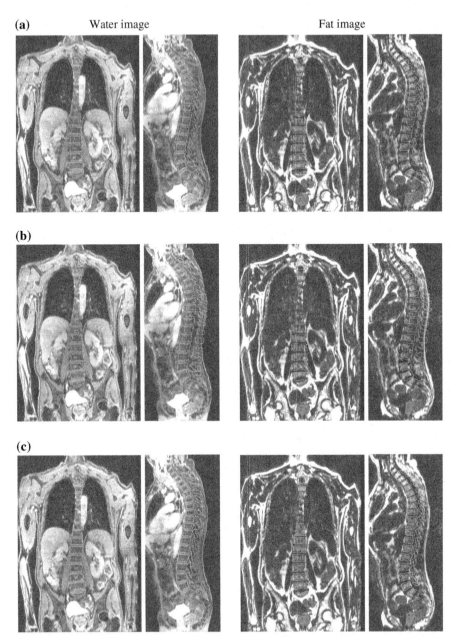

Fig. 4 Segmentation steps from *Pat2* using multi-modal features, overlaid onto the water (*left*) and the fat image (*right*). **a** Model localization. The complete model is positioned in the image. **b** Parametric adaptation. Multiple parametric transformations adapt the anchoring structures (*red*) to the image, while all vertebrae (*yellow*) are deactivated and passivly transformed to avoid wrong vertebra correspondences. **c** Deformable adaptation. The vertebrae are iteratively activated and adapted to the image (from sacrum to neck). This last step finalizes the segmentation

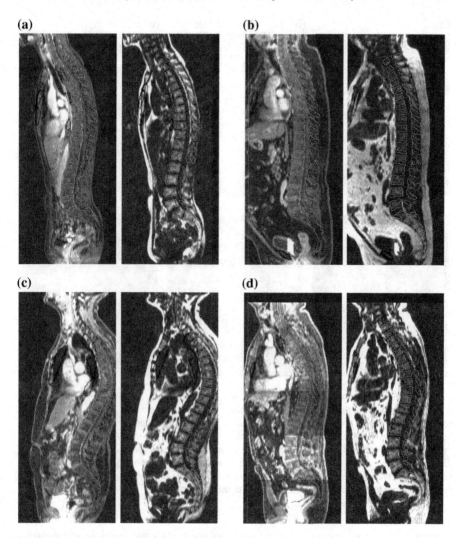

Fig. 5 Segmentation results from four patients, *Pat3* to *Pat6* (a–d), using the proposed multi-modal image features. For each patient, segmentation results are overlaid onto the water (*left*) as well as onto the fat image (*right*), in sagittal view only. All vertebrae were segmented correctly, with a maximum error of 1.81 mm for *Pat4*. As can be observed,, our method is robust against patient size (*Pat3* vs. *Pat4*), spine shape (*Pat4* vs. *Pat5*), and stitching artifacts (*Pat6*)

5 Discussion

In this paper we proposed a fully automatic model-based approach to segment the vertebrae from Dixon MR images. Our experiments showed that using a single image from the Dixon sequence alone (i.e. the water or fat image) might lead to large

(a)   **(b)** *Pat7* : Waterfailure   **(c)**

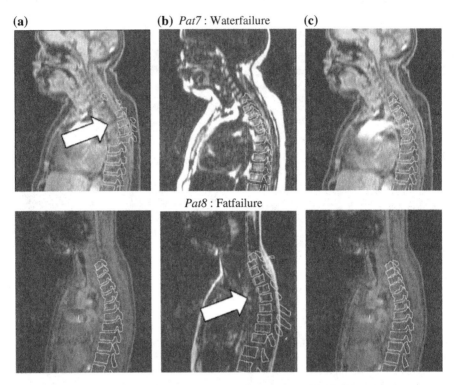

Pat8 : Fatfailure

Fig. 6 Segmentation comparison for two patients, *Pat7* (*top*) and *Pat8* (*bottom*), using **a** water features (overlaid onto the water image), **b** fat features (overlaid onto the fat image), **c** multi-modal features (only overlaid onto the water image here). For *Pat7*, segmentation using only the water image fails around the top thoracic vertebrae due to low image contrast (largest error of 14.27 mm in thoracic vertebra 4). For *Pat8*, segmentation using only the fat image again fails around the top thoracic vertebrae (larest error of 15.48 mm in thoracic vertebra 6). Segmentation using multi-modal features remains robust in both cases ((maximum error for *Pat7*: 4.00 mm (thoracic vertebra 5) maximum error for *Pat8*: 4.75 mm (thoracic vertebra 7))

segmentation errors due to varying image contrasts: in some cases image contrast between the vertebrae is better in the water image, in other cases contrast is better in the fat image. Our multi-modal feature approach uses both the water and the fat image simultaneously for segmentation. Considering all patients, the multi-modal features reduced the segmentation error from 2.89 mm (water)/2.11 mm (fat) to 1.69 mm, which is an improvement of up to 41 %. Our method provided accurate segmentation results for all of the 25 patients. It is robust against variations in patient size (comparing slim *Pat3* with big *Pat4*), against variations in the spine shape (comparing the straigt spine shape in *Pat4* with the curved shape in *Pat5*), as well as against stitching artifacts when combining images from multiple bed positions (horizontal streaks in *Pat6*).

Table 1 Validation of vertebra segmentations from all 25 patients

Anatomical region	Surface distances (mm)		
	Water features	Fat features	Multi-modal features
Thoracic vertebra 1	4.71 (36.32 %)	3.85 (25.58 %)	3.76 (24.87 %)
Thoracic vertebra 2	4.76 (29.06 %)	3.03 (18.21 %)	2.54 (11.44 %)
Thoracic vertebra 3	4.02 (28.33 %)	2.47 (12.60 %)	1.67 (4.55 %)
Thoracic vertebra 4	4.34 (31.33 %)	2.79 (14.01 %)	1.96 (6.85 %)
Thoracic vertebra 5	3.62 (25.86 %)	3.03 (15.05 %)	2.01 (8.29 %)
Thoracic vertebra 6	3.77 (25.05 %)	2.93 (13.23 %)	1.84 (6.79 %)
Thoracic vertebra 7	3.45 (23.99 %)	2.99 (14.21 %)	1.94 (7.81 %)
Thoracic vertebra 8	3.07 (17.03 %)	2.72 (13.19 %)	1.78 (6.31 %)
Thoracic vertebra 9	2.76 (12.56 %)	2.59 (13.69 %)	1.57 (4.24 %)
Thoracic vertebra 10	2.37 (8.87 %)	1.97 (8.10 %)	1.33 (1.12 %)
Thoracic vertebra 11	1.64 (4.23 %)	1.50 (3.27 %)	1.23 (0.19 %)
Thoracic vertebra 12	1.92 (5.28 %)	1.38 (1.35 %)	1.25 (0.77 %)
Lumbar vertebra 1	1.79 (4.83 %)	1.32 (1.52 %)	1.21 (1.35 %)
Lumbar vertebra 2	1.70 (4.39 %)	1.36 (2.73 %)	1.20 (1.80 %)
Lumbar vertebra 3	1.55 (4.12 %)	1.14 (0.31 %)	1.04 (0.32 %)
Lumbar vertebra 4	1.71 (4.04 %)	1.14 (0.41 %)	1.08 (0.25 %)
Lumbar vertebra 5	1.95 (4.93 %)	1.45 (2.86 %)	1.29 (0.87 %)
Whole spine	2.89 (15.90 %)	2.22 (9.43 %)	1.69 (5.17 %)

For each vertebra, mesh surface distances to the reference ground truth annotation as well as the amount of triangles showing an error of larger than 5 mm were computed. We compared segmentations using (a) water features, (b) fat features and (c) the proposed multi-modal (water and fat) image features. As can be observed, segmentations using water and fat features showed mean errors of 2.89 and 2.22 mm, respectively, while our multi-modal features achieved highest segmentation accuracy with a clear reduction to a mean error 1.69 mm (over all 17 vertabrae and all 25 patients), which is within the order of the image resolution ($0.8 \times 0.8 \times 3\ mm^3$)

In future work, the inclusion of more patients for training could improve the model. Large segmentation errors such as of the last thoracic vertebra 1 could be minimized, e.g. by including more prior shape knowledge into the segmentation pipeline. In our current approach, a mesh triangle is simultaneously attracted to a water and fat image target point, while both forces are equally weighted. Adaptive forces that attract the triangle to a target point depending on the underlying feature strength could further improve segmentation accuracy. Regarding computation times, a segmentation currently requires approximately 5–6 min on a 4-core notebook, Intel(R) Core(TM) CPUs at 2.6 GHz, 4 GB RAM memory. Hierarchical approaches using multi-resolution meshes (start segmentation on low resolution meshes and finalize on high resolution meshes) could be applied to minimize computation times.

Our current approach was used to derive a model-based segmentation from two input images (water and fat image). However, our approach can also be applied to more than two images. Alternative applications might be the segmentation of a diffusion image series or a dynamic contrast enhances image series to maximize image contrast and segmentation accuracy compared to only using a single image from the series.

The approach can be used in hybrid PET/MR imaging systems to include bone tissue in PET attenuation correction (AC) without the need of additional MR sequences for bone visualization, such as UTE. While the validation of this paper was focused on the segmentation of the vertebrae, we plan to validate the segmentation accuracy of the remaining model components. This will lead us to our overall goal of whole-body AC with five compartments (background, lung tissue, watery tissue, and fatty tissue, and bone tissue). Finally, the PET image could be included into the presented Dixon segmentation allowing us to derive a single segmentation from anatomical (Dixon MR) as well as functional (PET) contrasts.

6 Conclusion

In this paper we introduced a model-based sementation with multi-modal features to extract the vertebrae from Dixon MR images. We showed that it improves robustness and accuracy of segmentation. Our method can be considered for MR-based PET attenuation correction (including bone tissue as additional attenuation compartment). Further possible applications are computer-aided diagnosis of diseases such as spinal disc degeneration, automated spine scan planning, or image-guided interventions such as computer-assisted surgery.

Acknowledgments We thank Bénédicte Delattre and the Hôpitaux Universitaire de Genève, in particular Prof. Osman Ratib, for providing us with the Dixon MR image data.

References

1. Martinez-Moeller, A., Souvatzoglou, M., Delso, G., Bundschuh, R.A., Chefd'hotel, C., Ziegler, S.I., Navab, N., Schwaiger, M., Nekolla, S.G.: Tissue classification as a potential approach for attenuation correction in whole-body PET/MRI: evaluation with PET/CT data. J. Nuc. Med. **50**(4), 520–526 (2009)
2. Buerger, C., Tsoumpas, C., Aitken, A., King, A.P., Schleyer, P., Schulz, V., Marsden, P.K., Schaeffter, T.: Investigation of MR-Based attenuation correction and motion compensation for hybrid PET/MR. IEEE Trans. Nuc. Sci. **59**(5), 1967–1976 (2012)
3. Berker, Y., Franke, J., Salomon, A., Palmowski, M., Donker, H.C.W., Temur, Y., Mottaghy, F.M., Kuhl, C., Izquierdo-Garcia, D., Fayad, Z.A., Kiessling, F., Schulz, V.: MRI-Based attenuation correction for hybrid PET/MRI systems: a 4-class tissue segmentation technique using a combined ultrashort-echo-time/Dixon MRI sequence. J. Nuc. Med. **53**(5), 796–804 (2012)
4. Michopoulou, S., Costaridou, L., Panagiotopoulos, E., Speller, R., Panayiotakis, G., Todd-Pokropek, A.: Atlas-based segmentation of degenerated lumbar intervertebral discs from MR images of the spine. IEEE Trans. Biomed. Eng. **56**(9), 2225–2231 (2009)
5. Carballido-Gamio, J., Belongie, S., Majumdar, S.: Normalized cuts in 3-d for spinal MRI segmentation. IEEE Trans. Med. Imaging **23**(1), 36–44 (2004)
6. Michael Kelm, B., Wels, M., Kevin Zhou, S., Seifert, S., Suehling, M., Zheng, Y., Comaniciu, D.: Spine detection in CT and MR using iterated marginal space learning. Med. Image Anal. (2012)

7. Kadoury, S., Labelle, H., Paragios, N.: Spine segmentation in medical images using manifold embeddings and higher-order MRFs (2013)
8. Zhan, Y., Maneesh, D., Harder, M., Zhou, X.S.: Robust MR spine detection using hierarchical learning and local articulated model. In: Medical Image Computing and Computer-Assisted Intervention, pp. 141–148. Springer (2012)
9. Hoad, C.L., Martel, A.L.: Segmentation of MR images for computer-assisted surgery of the lumbar spine. Phys Med Biol **47**(19), 3503 (2002)
10. Ecabert, O., Peters, J., Schramm, H., Lorenz, C., von Berg, J., Walker, M., Vembar, M., Olszewski, M., Subramanyan, K., Lavi, G., Weese, J.: Automatic model-based segmentation of the heart in CT images. IEEE Trans. Med. Imaging **27**(9), 1189–1201 (2008)
11. Peters, J., Ecabert, O., Meyer, C., Kneser, R., Weese, J.: Optimizing boundary detection via simulated search with applications to multi-modal heart segmentation. Med. Image Anal. **14**(1), 70–84 (2010)

Segmentation of Lumbar Intervertebral Discs from High-Resolution 3D MR Images Using Multi-level Statistical Shape Models

Aleš Neubert, Jurgen Fripp, Craig Engstrom and Stuart Crozier

Abstract Three-dimensional (3D) high resolution magnetic resonance (MR) scans of the lumbar spine provide relevant diagnostic information for lumbar interverte-bral disc related disorders. Automated segmentation algorithms, such as active shape modelling, have the potential to facilitate the processing of the complex 3D MR data. An active shape model employs prior anatomical information about the segmented shapes that is typically described by standard principle component analysis. In this study, performance of this traditional statistical shape model was compared to that of a multi-level statistical shape model, incorporating the hierarchical structure of the spine. The mean Dice score coefficient, mean absolute square distance and Haus-dorff distance obtained with the multi-level model were significantly better than those obtained with the traditional shape model. These initial results warrant further investigation of potential benefits that the multi-level statistical shape models can have in spine image analysis.

A. Neubert (✉) · J. Fripp
The Australian E-Health Research Centre, CSIRO Computational Informatics,
Brisbane, Australia
e-mail: ales.neubert@uqconnect.edu.au

A. Neubert · S. Crozier
School of Information Technology and Electrical Engineering,
The University of Queensland, Brisbane, Australia
e-mail: stuart@itee.uq.edu.au

C. Engstrom
School of Human Movement Studies, The University of Queensland,
Brisbane, Australia
e-mail: craig@hms.uq.edu.au

J. Yao et al. (eds.), *Computational Methods and Clinical Applications*
for Spine Imaging, Lecture Notes in Computational Vision and Biomechanics 17,
DOI: 10.1007/978-3-319-07269-2_15, © Springer International Publishing Switzerland 2014

1 Introduction

Magnetic resonance (MR) imaging provides an excellent diagnostic tool for assessing common spine pathologies [3]. Traditional radiological spine exams consist of acquisition of several multi-slice two-dimensional (2D) MR scans, usually in sagittal and axial orientation. Recent advances in MR hardware, software and MR sequence design introduce new possibilities in musculoskeletal radiology by acquiring high resolution three-dimensional (3D) scans, for example using the SPACE MR sequence (3D Sampling Perfection with Application optimised Contrasts using different flip angle Evolution) [9]. These images enable more detailed 3D visualisation of the intervertebral discs (IVDs) and have demonstrated an increased sensitivity to several spine pathologies [10]. The high resolution and associated acquisition artefacts challenge post-processing procedures that are important to alleviate time- and expertise-intensive assessment in the context of clinical and applied research environments (anatomy segmentation or delineation of a region-of-interest, morphological assessment).

The capacity for MR imaging to provide high contrast scans of the IVDs is counterweighted by the fact that most current studies are acquired with anisotropic resolution. Hence previous segmentation approaches have been based on 2D analyses, typically based on images obtained in the sagittal plane. Several edge detecting techniques have been exploited to find the precise IVD boundaries, such as Hough transform [14]. Edge detectors are combined with a trained classifier based on statistical textural features to distinguish clusters of the IVDs by Chevrefils et al. [1]. The Generalised Hough Transform is used in the segmentation pipeline of Seifert et al. [13], followed by active contours driven active shape model (ASM) segmentation, progressing in neighbouring transversal slices. The segmentation results from all slices are appended into final 3D volume. A combination of fuzzy c-means technique with prior knowledge from a probabilistic disc atlas was presented by Michopoulou et al. [11] to segment discs in a mid-sagittal slice.

To the best of our knowledge, all previous approaches have been segmenting the IVDs from 2D slices, employing 2D segmentation techniques. In our recent work, we presented an automated 3D segmentation of the IVDs from high-resolution MR data, based on standard 3D active shape models and grey level profile modelling [12]. In the current study, we evaluate the multi-level statistical shape models (MSSM) of Lecron et al. [7] in an automated segmentation of lumbar IVDs from high-resolution MR scans. It was suggested by Lecron et al. [7] that these models are more suitable to describe hierarchical structures (as the human spine), and were successfully applied to reconstruction of vertebrae from bi-planar radiographs [8]. The segmentation of IVDs from MR images presented in this work slightly adapts the MSSM that model within-class and between-class variations in 3D shapes of lumbar IVDs and combines them with a statistical shape models (SSM) of coarse global shape variation of the lumbar spine. These models are used in a segmentation task to automatically delineate the lumbar IVDs, and compared against a traditional SSM. The aim of this study is to test whether the performance of the automated segmentation can be improved with the MSSM and to motivate its further use in automated 3D analysis of IVDs from high resolution MR images.

2 Method

2.1 Image Database

MR scans of the lumbar spine of 12 subjects (9 male, 3 female) were acquired using the 3D T2-weighted SPACE pulse sequence at 3T Siemens Trio MR system. This protocol has good potential for clinical assessment and diagnosis [9, 10], has the advantage of 3D volumetric acquisition and provides high-resolution images with superior level of details (axial slice thickness 1–1.2 mm, in-plane resolution 0.34 × 0.34 mm). Two scans of each subject were acquired and stitched together to cover all lumbar IVDs from T12/L1 to L4/L5. The acquisition time was 7 min 50 s per block.

Although all 12 subjects were 'asymptomatic' healthy volunteers, disc degeneration was observed in 4 subject (6/60 lumbar IVDs) by a trained radiologist. Such abnormal findings are common in the asymptomatic population and are in accordance with numbers reported in previous clinical studies [5]. Other radiological findings included vertebral haemangiomas in 2 cases and several Schmorl's nodes (vertebral endplate fracture) of varying dimensions.

All cases were manually segmented and used to generate the statistical shape models and to quantitatively evaluate the segmentation algorithm.

The medical research ethics committee of the University of Queensland approved the current study and written informed consent was obtained from all participants involved.

2.2 Image Pre-processing

Two slightly overlapping serial blocks were acquired for each subject in this study and stitched together using a customised algorithm explained in more details in [12]. The pre-processing steps further included an intensity inhomogeneity correction based on the N4 bias field correction algorithm [16], smoothing by gradient anisotropic diffusion (15 iterations with time step 0.01 and conductivity 0.25) and signal intensity value standardisation by atlas matching of the image histograms extracted from the spinal column.

2.3 *Image Segmentation*

The segmentation algorithm is based on the method of active shape models (ASM) [2]. The ASM is initialised by a series of object recognition techniques as presented in [12]. This method estimates the spine curve and detects centres of vertebral bodies. The initial IVD models are placed half way between detected vertebral bodies and oriented to follow the estimated spine curve. The algorithm was successful in detecting 58/60 vertebral bodies. In 2 cases, the lower-most vertebral body L5 was missed and annotated manually.

This section outlines the traditional and the multi-level statistical shape models, presents the segmentation scheme and parameters, and explains the validation procedure.

2.3.1 Traditional Statistical Shape Models

After initial shape alignment (the generalised Procrustes alignment [6]), a point distribution can be defined for the positions of spatially corresponding shape vertices $x_i^j \in \mathbb{R}^3$ for $i \in \{1, \ldots, N\}$ shapes consisting of $j \in \{1, \ldots, J\}$ vertices. The mean shape $\bar{x}$ and covariance matrix C are computed. Each shape S_i is represented as an n-dimensional vector $\mathbf{x_i}$. The shape vectors can be represented in the form of:

$$\mathbf{x_i} = \bar{\mathbf{x}} + \mathbf{Pb_i} = \bar{\mathbf{x}} + \sum_{m=1}^{N} \mathbf{p}^m b_i^m$$

where $\mathbf{P} = \{\mathbf{p}^m | m = 1, \ldots, N\}$ are the eigenvectors of the covariance matrix C (with corresponding eigenvalues $\{\lambda^m | m = 1, \ldots, N\}$) and $\mathbf{b_i} = \{b_i^m | m = 1, \ldots, N\}$ are the weights of each mode of variation (also called shape parameters) parameterising the shape S_i. The number of used modes of variation is usually reduced since a smaller number of modes $n < N$ can explain most variation in the dataset.

One statistical shape model from all lumbar discs was generated. The point correspondences were obtained using SPHARM parameterisation and groupwise optimisation of the description length [4].

2.3.2 Multi-level Statistical Shape Model

The MSSM presented by Lecron et al. [7] applies principles of multi-level component analysis [15] to describe variations in hierarchical structures. In the example of the lumbar spine in this study, the structure of $N = 60$ intervertebral discs is divided into $K = 5$ groups of disc levels (T12/L1 to L4/L5) where each groups consists of 12 discs of the same level of different subjects. The multi-level component analysis finds independent components of within-class and between-class variation from a

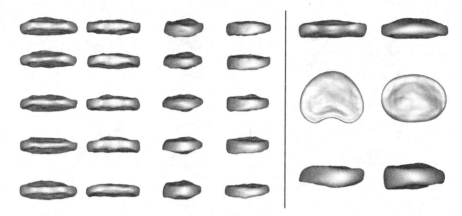

Fig. 1 Modes of variation of the multi-level statistical model. First mode of the within-class component is shown in the *left panel* (posterior and lateral views). The mode primarily captures a relative IVD narrowing (inferior–superior). The first mode of the between-class component is shown in the *right panel* (posterior, superior and lateral views). The mode describes anterior–posterior wedging and changes from a circular to a 'bean' like shape. These are typical differences between inferior and superior lumbar IVDs

decomposition of each shape belonging to a group k as:

$$^{\mathbf{k}}\mathbf{x}_i = \bar{\mathbf{x}} + (^{\mathbf{k}}\bar{\mathbf{x}} - \bar{\mathbf{x}}) + (^{\mathbf{k}}\mathbf{x}_i - ^{\mathbf{k}}\bar{\mathbf{x}}),$$

where $^{\mathbf{k}}\bar{\mathbf{x}}$ is the mean shape of class k. This decomposition defines two-level hierarchical model where the within-class variation (same IVD level) and between-class variation are modelled independently.

A lumbar spine $\mathbf{X_i} = \{^{\mathbf{k}}\mathbf{x}_i | k \in 1, \ldots, K\}$ can be reconstructed from the components of within-class variation $\mathbf{P}^w$ and the between-class variation $\mathbf{P}^b$:

$$\mathbf{X}_i = \begin{pmatrix} ^1\mathbf{x}_i \\ \vdots \\ ^K\mathbf{x}_i \end{pmatrix} = \begin{pmatrix} \bar{\mathbf{x}} \\ \vdots \\ \bar{\mathbf{x}} \end{pmatrix} + \begin{pmatrix} \mathbf{b}_i^w \\ \vdots \\ \mathbf{b}_i^w \end{pmatrix} \mathbf{P}^w + \begin{pmatrix} ^1\mathbf{b}_i^b \\ \vdots \\ ^K\mathbf{b}_i^b \end{pmatrix} \mathbf{P}^b,$$

where $\mathbf{b}_i^w$ and $^k\mathbf{b}_i^b$, $k \in \{1, \ldots, K\}$ are respectively the within-class and between-class shape parameters for the spine $\mathbf{X}_i$. The within-class component describes global anatomical differences between individual subjects, whereas the between-class component describes changes between IVDs at different levels of the lumbar spine (from T12/L1 to L4/L5). As such, both components are important for a successful segmentation. The most important modes of variation are presented in Fig. 1.

In contrast to Lecron et al. [7], all shapes are initially aligned (the generalised Procrustes alignment [6]) and the MSSM do not contain any information on relative poses of the IVDs, allowing to model uniquely the variation in shape. We model the coarse global variation in relative disc positions and their scale by a simplified

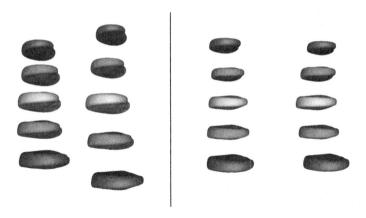

Fig. 2 General model of coarse variation of the lumbar spine. The first mode (*left*) describes the extension of the lumbar spine and some relative changes in the IVD size. The second mode (*right*) describes primarily the extent of the lordosis. For visualisation purposes, the statistical mean shape was inserted to the locations described by the coarse model and scaled accordingly

statistical model. A $K \times 4$ matrix containing the centroid points of each IVD and its scale (in each row) is constructed for every lumbar spine and the principle component analysis is performed. This analysis is used as a rough control over the global shape of the segmented spine and allows the MSSM to focus on changes between individual shapes. The first two modes of the global lumbar spine variation are shown in Fig. 2.

2.3.3 Shape Deformation

The shape deformation procedure is an iterative process driven by grey level profile matching. Initially, training profiles are extracted from the manually segmented shapes in the database. At each iteration, grey level profiles $\hat{\mathbf{p}}^j$ of lengths $2R + 1 > 2L + 1$ (length of the training profiles) are extracted along the normals for each vertex v^j, $j = 1, \ldots, J$ of the positioned shape V. The spacing h is the same for both the training and matching profiles and all profiles are normalised to zero mean and unit variance. The displacement of each vertex is determined by first extracting sub-profiles $\hat{\mathbf{p}}^{j,r}$, $r = 1, \ldots, 1 + R - L$ of length $2L + 1$ from $\hat{\mathbf{p}}^j$ by moving the profile centre point. All profiles are compared to all training profiles $\mathbf{p}_i^j$, $i = 1, \ldots, N$ of the corresponding vertex v^j by evaluating the normalised cross-correlation (NCC) similarity metric to determine the optimal displacement along the vertex normal. The new position is determined as the centre of the sub-profile $\hat{\mathbf{p}}^{j,r_{max}}$ maximising the NCC across all possible displacements from all corresponding profiles:

$$\hat{\mathbf{p}}^{j,r_{max}} \leftarrow \arg\max_{i,r} NCC(\hat{\mathbf{p}}^{j,r}, \mathbf{p}_i^j)$$

Table 1 Numerical values of used parameters

Parameter	Connotation	Value
n	Number of modes for the traditional SSM	8
n^b	Number of between-class modes for the MSSM	10
n^w	Number of within-class modes for the MSSM	2
	Number of iterations for both ASM	100
$2L+1$	Points in training profiles	61
h	Profile spacing (mm)	0.25
$2R+1$	Points in matching profiles	81
b_{max}	Shape constraint for all shape models	2.0

After every iteration, the overall shape deformation is restrained by the modes of variation of the corresponding statistical shape model to preserve the anatomical validity of the segmented shape.

2.4 Algorithm Setup and Parameters

Both active shape models were applied to segment lumbar IVDs from 12 subjects and evaluated against the manual reference. The IVDs were segmented independently (in parallel) when using the traditional SSM, whereas a simultaneous segmentation of the whole set of lumbar IVDs is necessary for the MSSM, since the multi-level component analysis is applied to the whole lumbar spine section composed of 5 IVDs. No further post-processing steps were performed.

The algorithm parameters are presented in Table 1. The number of modes used in every shape model was chosen to comprise 90 % of the total variation and the shape constraints were applied after every iteration. The segmentation was run for 100 iterations, however this number was not optimised. The global shape constraints defining the relative positions and scale of the lumbar IVDs was applied every 5th iteration during the first 50 iterations to increase the robustness to initialisation.

2.5 Evaluation

The Dice score coefficient (DSC), the mean absolute square distance (MASD) and the Hausdorff distance were used as similarity measures. The accuracy metrics for the traditional SSM were computed using the segmentation results from [12], evaluated on the 12 cases used in this study. Student's t-test for independent samples were used

Table 2 Statistics of the segmentation results (* significantly different)

Measure	Traditional SSM	Multi-level SSM
DSC (mean $\pm$ StDev)	0.898 ± 0.027	$0.911 \pm 0.025*$
DSC (median)	0.902	0.915
DSC (minimum)	0.805	0.818
MASD (mean $\pm$ StDev)	0.56 ± 0.14	$0.48 \pm 0.16*$
MASD (median)	0.54	0.47
MASD (maximum)	1.00	1.02
Hausdorff (mean $\pm$ StDev)	3.64 ± 1.08	$3.15 \pm 1.12*$
Hausdorff (median)	3.58	2.83
Hausdorff (maximum)	7.20	6.91

to compare the mean values between segmentation results obtained with traditional and multi-level SSM. The level of significance was set at $p < 0.05$.

3 Results

The performance of both active shape models in IVD segmentation can be viewed in Table 2 and Fig. 3. The mean DSC obtained with the MSSM were significantly higher than those obtained with the traditional SSM (0.911 ± 0.025 vs. 0.898 ± 0.027, $p = 0.007$). Similarly, significantly better performance of the MSSM measured by the MASD (0.48 ± 0.16 mm vs. 0.56 ± 0.14 mm, $p = 0.005$) and the Hausdorff distance (3.15 ± 1.12 mm vs. 3.64 ± 1.08 mm, $p = 0.017$) was observed compared to the traditional SSM. An example of the performance of both models is provided in Fig. 4, highlighting some improvements delivered by the MSSM.

Two-dimensional segmentation of the IVDs in sagittal slices have been previously achieved with DSC 0.85 for scoliotic spines [1], or DSC 0.92 and MASD 0.98 px = 0.613 mm [11]. Seifert et al. [13] combines the 2D IVD segmentation into volumes achieving DSC between 0.84 and 0.98, MASD between 1.19 and 1.61 px translating to 1.86–2.5 mm and Hausdorff distance between 2.00 and 4.24 px or 3.12–6.62 mm. Lower MASD of our method is possible due to both the algorithm accuracy and the high resolution database. To the best of our knowledge, there is no intrinsically 3D approach enabling direct comparison. The comparison between 2D and 3D segmentation techniques is challenging because of the different acquisition parameters and nature of used images (with higher inter-slice gap).

The results suggest that the MSSM contains relevant information about the morphology of the lumbar IVDs and that the multi-level spine modelling have the potential to improve segmentation accuracy. Extended validation is essential to confirm

Fig. 3 *Box plots* presenting the validation metrics. The numerical statistics can be found in Table 2

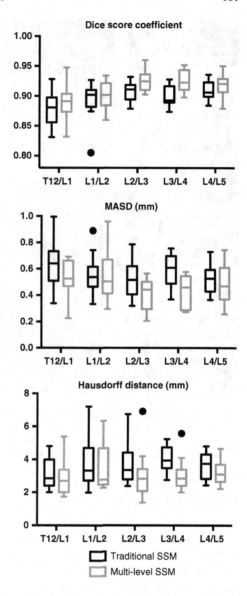

this initial results and to test the ability of both models to segment IVDs with various pathologies. Future work will also include evaluation of the robustness of both models to initialisation, that is crucial for implementation in large scale studies.

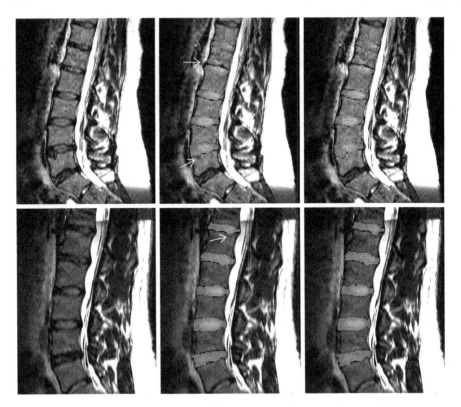

Fig. 4 Example cases with overlaid segmentations obtained with the traditional (*middle*) and multi-level (*right*) shape model. The manual segmentation is shown in *green*, the automatic in *red* and their overlay in *yellow*. Some areas where the MSSM improves the results are noted with *arrows*, including two Schmorl's nodes (*bottom arrow* in the *upper image*, *arrow* in the *lower image*)

4 Conclusion

Active shape models are well suited for segmentation of intervertebral discs from high resolution MR images. The performance is dependant on the ability of the underlying statistical shape model to capture and model natural variation of the segmented anatomy. A traditional statistical shape model of lumbar intervertebral discs was compared to a multi-level statistical shape model, describing hierarchical structure of the lumbar spine, in automated MR segmentation. Significantly better performance of the multi-level shape model warrants further investigation of its potential application in spine image analysis.

Acknowledgments The authors would like to thank Dr. Duncan Walker for the radiological assessments. This research was supported under Australian Research Council's linkage project funding scheme LP100200422.

References

1. Chevrefils, C., Chériet, F., Aubin, C.E., Grimard, G.: Texture analysis for automatic segmentation of intervertebral disks of scoliotic spines from MR images. IEEE Trans. Inf. Technol. Biomed. **13**(4), 608–620 (2009)
2. Cootes, T.F., Taylor, C.J., Cooper, D.H., Graham, J.: Active shape models-their training and application. Comput. Vis. Image Underst. **61**(1), 38–59 (1995)
3. Cousins, J.P., Haughton, V.M.: Magnetic resonance imaging of the spine. J. Am. Acad. Orthop. Surg. **17**(1), 22–30 (2009)
4. Davies, R.H., Twining, C.J., Taylor, C.: Groupwise surface correspondence by optimization: representation and regularization. Med. Image Anal. **12**(6), 787–796 (2008)
5. Emch, T.M., Modic, M.T.: Imaging of lumbar degenerative disk disease: history and current state. Skelet. Radiol. **40**(9), 1175–1189 (2011)
6. Gower, J.C.: Generalized procrustes analysis. Psychometrika **40**(1), 33–51 (1975)
7. Lecron, F., Boisvert, J., Benjelloun, M., Labelle, H., Mahmoudi, S.: Multilevel statistical shape models : a new framework for modeling hierarchical structures. In: International Symposium on Biomedical Imaging: From Nano to Macro, pp. 1284–1287 (2012)
8. Lecron, F., Boisvert, J., Mahmoudi, S., Labelle, H., Benjelloun, M.: Fast 3D Spine Reconstruction of Postoperative Patients Using a Multilevel Statistical Model. In: International Conference on Medical Image Computing and Computer-Assisted Intervention (MICCAI) **15**, 446–453 (2012)
9. Lichy, M.P., Wietek, B.M., Mugler, J.P., Horger, W., Menzel, M.I., Anastasiadis, A., Siegmann, K., Niemeyer, T., Königsrainer, A., Kiefer, B., Schick, F., Claussen, C.D., Schlemmer, H.P.: Magnetic resonance imaging of the body trunk using a single-slab, 3-dimensional, T2-weighted turbo-spin-echo sequence with high sampling efficiency (SPACE) for high spatial resolution imaging: initial clinical experiences. Invest. Radiol. **40**(12), 754–760 (2005)
10. Meindl, T., Wirth, S., Weckbach, S., Dietrich, O., Reiser, M., Schoenberg, S.O.: Magnetic resonance imaging of the cervical spine: comparison of 2D T2-weighted turbo spin echo, 2D T2*weighted gradient-recalled echo and 3D T2-weighted variable flip-angle turbo spin echo sequences. Eur. Radiol. **19**(3), 713–721 (2009)
11. Michopoulou, S.K., Costaridou, L., Panagiotopoulos, E., Speller, R., Panayiotakis, G., Todd-Pokropek, A.: Atlas-based segmentation of degenerated lumbar intervertebral discs from MR images of the spine. IEEE Trans. Biomed. Eng. **56**(9), 2225–2231 (2009)
12. Neubert, A., Fripp, J., Engstrom, C., Schwarz, R., Lauer, L., Salvado, O., Crozier, S.: Automated detection, 3D segmentation and analysis of high resolution spine MR images using statistical shape models. Phys. Med. Biol. **57**(24), 8357–8376 (2012)
13. Seifert, S., Wachter, I., Schmelzle, G., Dillmann, R.: A knowledge-based approach to soft tissue reconstruction of the cervical spine. IEEE Trans. Med. Imaging **28**(4), 494–507 (2009)
14. Shi, R., Sun, D., Qiu, Z., Weiss, K.L.: An efficient method for segmentation of MRI spine images. In: IEEE: International Conference on Complex Medical, Engineering, pp. 713–717 (2007)
15. Timmerman, M.E.: Multilevel component analysis. Br. J. Math. Stat. Pychol. **59**(Pt 2), 301–320 (2006)
16. Tustison, N.J., Gee, J.C.: N4ITK: nicks N3 ITK implementation for MRI bias field correction. Insight J. **2009**, 1–8 (2009)

A Supervised Approach Towards Segmentation of Clinical MRI for Automatic Lumbar Diagnosis

Subarna Ghosh, Manavender R. Malgireddy,
Vipin Chaudhary and Gurmeet Dhillon

Abstract Lower back pain (LBP) is widely prevalent in people all over the world. It is associated with chronic pain and change in posture which negatively affects our quality of life. Automatic segmentation of intervertebral discs and the dural sac along with labeling of the discs from clinical lumbar MRI is the first step towards computer-aided diagnosis of lower back ailments like desiccation, herniation and stenosis. In this paper we propose a supervised approach to simultaneously segment the vertebra, intervertebral discs and the dural sac of clinical sagittal MRI using the neighborhood information of each pixel. Experiments on 53 cases out of which 40 were used for training and the rest for testing, show encouraging Dice Similarity Indices of 0.8483 and 0.8160 for the dural sac and intervertebral discs respectively.

1 Introduction

Lower back pain is the second most common neurological ailment in the United States after headache [5] with more than $50 billion spent annually on rehabilitation and healthcare. In the past decade there has been a severe shortage of radiologists [2] and projections show that by the year 2020 there will be a significant boom in the ratio of their demand and supply. This concern motivates us to automatically detect and diagnose various lumbar abnormalities from clinical scans to reduce the average time for diagnosis and help to curtail excessive burden on radiologists.

S. Ghosh (✉) · M. R. Malgireddy · V. Chaudhary
Department of Computer Science and Engineering, State University of New York (SUNY)
at Buffalo, Buffalo, NY 14260, USA
e-mail: sghosh7@buffalo.edu

G. Dhillon
Proscan Imaging Inc., Williamsville, NY 14221, USA
e-mail: gdhillon@gmail.com

J. Yao et al. (eds.), *Computational Methods and Clinical Applications*
for Spine Imaging, Lecture Notes in Computational Vision and Biomechanics 17,
DOI: 10.1007/978-3-319-07269-2_16, © Springer International Publishing Switzerland 2014

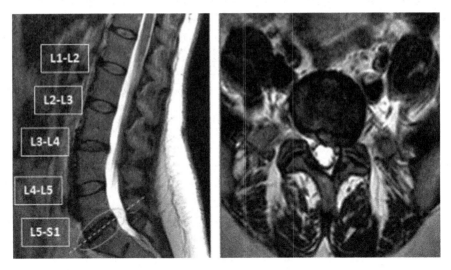

Fig. 1 (*Left*) Sagittal view of a lumbar MRI showing an L5-S1 disc herniation and (*Right*) the corresponding axial view of the lumbar MRI confirming a left sided herniation

CT and MRI are two popular modalities used to diagnose causes of lower back pain. While on one hand MRI is more expensive, it is non-invasive and also much better in terms of soft tissue detailing. Figure 1 illustrates intervertebral disc herniation diagnosed via the sagittal and axial slices of lumbar MRI. Requirements for CAD systems of the lumbar region are unique since we need to segment the dural sac and/or localize, label and segment the lumbar intervertebral discs before we can diagnose any abnormalities.

The lumbar vertebrae are the five vertebrae between the rib cage and the pelvis which are designated L1–L5, starting at the top. The lumbar vertebrae help support the weight of the body and permit movement. The intervertebral discs are fibrocartilaginous cushions serving as the spine's shock absorbing system, which protect the vertebrae, brain, and other structures. They are named depending on the vertebral bodies above and below, e.g., the disc in between L1 and L2 is named L1-L2 and so on. Dural sac is the membranous sac that encases the spinal cord within the bony structure of the vertebral column as shown in Fig. 2. The human spinal cord extends from the foramen magnum and continues through to the conus medullaris near the second lumbar vertebra, terminating in a fibrous extension known as the filum terminale. The dural sac usually ends at the vertebral level of the second sacral vertebra.

In general, MRI scans are very difficult to segment, since they suffer from partial volume effects and bias fields which might blur the delineation between different kinds of tissues. Moreover, localization of lumbar discs is a challenging problem due to a wide range of variabilities in the size, shape, count and appearance of discs and vertebrae. Similarly accurately segmenting the dural sac is also difficult due to variations in grayscale values and distortion in shape due to various abnormalities

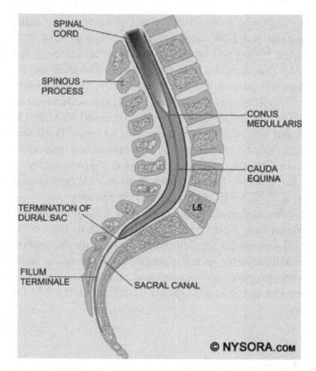

Fig. 2 This figure illustrates a cross section of the lumbar vertebrae and spinal cord. The position of the conus medullaris, cauda equina, termination of the dural sac and filum terminale are shown

like stenosis. To this end we propose an automatic method to simultaneously segment the vertebra, intervertebral discs and the dural sac of clinical sgittal MRI using the neighborhood information of each pixel. In the subsequent sections, we discuss in detail previous research (Sect. 2), our approach (Sect. 3) and experimental results (Sect. 4). Finally we draw our conclusion and discuss the scope for future work in Sect. 5.

2 Related Work

There has been quite some research in the direction of automatic dural sac segmentation [9–11], labeling and localization of intervertebral discs [1, 3, 8, 13, 14] and diagnosis of abnormalities [7] from lumbar MRI.

Schmidt et al. [14] introduced a probabilistic inference method using a part-based model that measures the possible locations of the intervertebral discs in full back MRI. They achieve upto 97 % part detection rate on 30 cases. Bhole et al. [3] presented a method for automatic detection of lumbar vertebrae and discs from clinical MRI by combining tissue property and geometric information from T1W sagittal, T2W sagittal and T2W axial modalities. They achieve 98.8 % accuracy for disc labeling on 67 sagittal images. Alomari et al. [1] proposed a two-level probabilistic model that captures both pixel- and object-level features to localize discs. The authors use generalized EM (Expectation Maximization) attaining an accuracy of 89.1 % on 50 test cases. Oktay et al. [13] proposed another approach using PHOG(pyramidal histogram of oriented gradients) based SVM and a probabilistic graphical model and achieved 95 % accuracy on 40 cases. In all these works, the authors have concentrated on localizing the vertebrae and/or intervertebral discs, i.e. they provide a point within the structure. Ghosh et al. [8] presented another approach using heuristics and machine learning methods to provide tight bounding boxes for each disc achieving 99 % localization accuracy on 53 cases.

Koh et al. [10] presented an automatic method for the segmentation of the dural sac using Gradient Vector Flow Field which achieved a similarity index of 0.7 on 52 cases. Horsfield et al. [9] proposed a semi-automatic method for the segmentation of the spinal cord from MRI utilizing an active surface model to assess multiple sclerosis. Koh et al. [11] also proposed an unsupervised and fully automatic method based on an attention model and an active contour model, achieving 0.71 Dice Similarity Index on 60 cases.

3 Proposed Approach

In most of the previous work, segmentation of the dural sac and the intervertebral discs have been handled separately which might lead to overlapping tissue regions. Moreover, some techniques depend on shape models which might lead to errors in case of high variability in appearance. Hence, in our proposed method, we adopt a unified approach where we simultaneously label each pixel as belonging to one of four class labels (vertebra, intervertebral disc, dural sac or background) using a probabilistic atlas and two decision trees based on the neighborhood information of each pixel.

3.1 Our Clinical Dataset

Clinical lumbar MRI used by our group is procured using a 3T Philips MRI scanner at Proscan Imaging Inc. It consists of manually co-registered T2 and T1 weighted sagittal views and T2 weighted axial views. We randomly pick 53 anonymized cases, all of which have one or more lumbar disc abnormalities. According to the radiologist's report there are a total of 65 herniated discs, 27 bulging discs, 26 desiccated discs, 60 degenerated discs and 73 disc levels having mild to severe stenosis.

For our experiments we use the T2 weighted mid-sagittal slice, each image having a resolution of 512×512. We use our own labeling tool for manual segmentation,

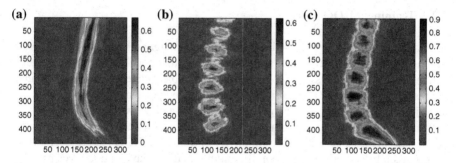

Fig. 3 Probabilistic Atlas of the lumbar region: **a**, **b** and **c** shows the atlas for the dural sac, the intervertebral discs and the vertebra respectively

which performs B-spline interplolation to interactively give a smooth outline of segmented regions, as shown in Figs. 4b and 5b. We randomly select 40 cases for training and the rest is kept aside for testing.

Let us denote $X = \{x_i : i \in \{1, 2, \ldots, n\}\}$ as the set of pixel grayscale values in the mid-sagittal image. Our approach treats the segmentation of lumbar MRI as a 4-class problem where each pixel can belong to any one of the following categories: vertebra, intervertebral disc, dural sac and background. The class labels are denoted by the set $L = \{l : l \in \{1, 2, 3, 4\}\}$ and the set of pixel labels $Y = \{y_i : i \in \{1, 2, \ldots, n\}, y_i \in \{L\}\}$ where y_i is the output class label for the ith pixel.

3.2 Training Phase

The training phase consists of the following three steps.

3.2.1 Creation of a Probabilistic Atlas

We create a simple probabilistic atlas (probability map) by combining the label information from manual segmentation of the 40 training images as illustrated in Fig. 3. Since the vetebral column is centrally located in the 512×512 image, we avoid a registration step which can be complicated due to high variability in intensities and shapes of structures in the lumbar region. The atlas is thus a $r \times c \times 4$ matrix where r and c are the total num of rows and columns respectively and $n = r \times c$ is the total number of pixels. Thus the probabilistic atlas gives us : $P_{atlas_i} \propto P(y_i = l | row_i, col_i)$ where l is the class label assigned to the ith pixel and (row_i, col_i) gives the location of the ith pixel in the image.

3.2.2 Training a HOG Tree

We train a classification tree [4] based on a pixel's neighborhood HOG(Histogram of Oriented Gradients) [6]. HOG are feature descriptors popularly used in computer vision and image processing for the purpose of object detection. This technique counts occurrences of gradient orientation in localized portions of an image. For our experiments, given an $h \times w$ neighborhood around a pixel, we divide it into 3×3 = 9 sub-windows and fix the bin size to 9 resulting in a vector of length 81. We empirically fix $h = w = 27$ and train the HOG tree using HOG feature vectors and pixel class labels obtained from our 40 training images. The hog tree gives us :

$$P_{hogTree_i} \propto P(y_i = l | hog_{nhood_i}),$$

where hog_{nhood_i} is the HOG calculated from the 27×27 image neighborhood around the ith pixel.

3.2.3 Training a Label Tree

We train another classification tree [4] based on a pixel's 27×27 neighborhood class labels. Hence the feature length is $27 \times 27 - 1 = 728$. The label tree gives us :

$$P_{labelTree_i} \propto P(y_i = l | label_{nhood_i}),$$

where $label_{nhood_i}$ is the class label information of the 27×27 neighborhood around the ith pixel.

3.3 Testing Phase

We implement two methods to segment our 13 test images.

3.3.1 Method 1

In this maximum-likelihood method we assign a class label to each pixel according to its location in the image (using the probabilistic atlas) and its neighborhood HOG information (using the HOG Tree). Mathematically, given a new image we assign a class label to each pixel as :

$$y_i = \underset{l}{\operatorname{argmax}} P(y_i = l | nhood_i),$$

where $P(y_i = l | nhood_i) \propto P_{hogTree_i} * P_{atlas_i}$.

3.3.2 Method 2

In this method we assign a class label to each pixel according to its location in the image (using the probabilistic atlas), its neighborhood HOG information (using the HOG tree) and its neighborhood label information (using the label tree). Given a new image we randomly assign a class label to each pixel and then utilise Gibbs sampling to sample a label for each pixel given its neighborhood HOG feature vector and all the other pixel labels. The update equation used is as follows:

$$P(y_i | nhood_i, \neg y_i) \propto (P_{hogTree_i} * P_{atlas_i} * P_{labelTree_i}).$$

We run Gibbs sampling for 200 iterations and use the last 100 iterations to decide the final class label, i.e. allow 100 iterations as burn in period.

3.3.3 Morphological Post-Processing

We finally apply binary morphological post-processing operations like closing, opening and hole filling on the resulting label maps to generate smoother segmentations.

4 Experimental Results

We use the Dice Coefficient as a Similarity Index to evaluate the validity of the automatic segmentation results. The Dice Coefficient $D(G, M)$ is defined as the ratio of twice the intersection over the sum of the two segmented results, the gold standard G and our automated result M :

$$Dice(G, M) = \frac{2 * n\{G \cap M\}}{n\{G\} + n\{M\}},$$

where $n\{G\}$ is the number of elements in set G. This measure is derived from a reliability measure known as the kappa (κ) statistic to evaluate the inter-observer agreement in regard to categorical data. According to this $D > 0.8$ indicates near-perfect agreement and $0.6 < D \leq 0.8$ represents substantial agreement and $0.4 < D \leq 0.6$ moderate agreement [12].

Tables 1 and 2 tabulate the Dice Similarity Indices of our automatic segmentation with respect to the expert manual segmentation. Table 1 lists the indices achieved by the two methods before morphological post-processing and Table 2 shows the indices after post-processing. We observe that the average results before post-processing fall in the category of 'substantial agreement', while after morphological operations the result indicates 'near-perfect agreement'. While Method 1 depends on the post-processing stage for its enhanced performance, before post-processing Method 2 (Gibbs Sampling) performs better than Method 1 since neighborhood label informa-

Table 1 Results: dice similarity indices before morphological post-processing

Case num	Method 1			Method 2 (Gibbs)		
	Dural sac	Disc	Vertebra	Dural sac	Disc	Vertebra
1	0.8203	0.6490	0.5730	0.8375	0.7271	0.8046
2	0.7949	0.6754	0.6784	0.8291	0.7622	0.8302
3	0.8245	0.6960	0.6934	0.8597	0.7938	0.8494
4	0.6467	0.5465	0.6401	0.6494	0.6136	0.8041
5	0.6918	0.4535	0.5961	0.6735	0.4716	0.6962
6	0.8136	0.6971	0.7004	0.8523	0.7799	0.8052
7	0.8312	0.5691	0.5897	0.8419	0.6189	0.7880
8	0.7436	0.6051	0.5676	0.7856	0.6804	0.7673
9	0.7506	0.5950	0.6069	0.7033	0.6431	0.7968
10	0.7433	0.6695	0.6280	0.8025	0.7803	0.7944
11	0.7416	0.6945	0.6948	0.7463	0.7510	0.7431
12	0.7710	0.5896	0.5740	0.8170	0.6769	0.7378
13	0.7024	0.6990	0.6863	0.6810	0.7689	0.8181
Avg	0.7597	0.6261	0.6330	0.7753	0.6975	0.7873

Table 2 Results: dice similarity indices after morphological post-processing

Case num	Method 1			Method 2 (Gibbs)		
	Dural sac	Disc	Vertebra	Dural sac	Disc	Vertebra
1	0.8765	0.8324	0.6853	0.8765	0.8023	0.8350
2	0.8881	0.8608	0.8130	0.8907	0.8595	0.8713
3	0.9107	0.8672	0.8329	0.9088	0.8703	0.8892
4	0.7419	0.7112	0.8197	0.7070	0.6849	0.8621
5	0.7844	0.5972	0.7166	0.7371	0.5704	0.7446
6	0.8985	0.8663	0.8644	0.9028	0.8533	0.8894
7	0.8960	0.7811	0.7245	0.8824	0.7362	0.8324
8	0.8427	0.8091	0.7284	0.8411	0.7955	0.8161
9	0.8522	0.7912	0.7934	0.7671	0.7532	0.8571
10	0.8272	0.8844	0.8071	0.8530	0.8728	0.8490
11	0.8090	0.9006	0.8731	0.7829	0.8479	0.8295
12	0.8843	0.8310	0.7700	0.8848	0.8165	0.8108
13	0.8167	0.8762	0.8444	0.7545	0.8530	0.8797
Avg	0.8483	0.8160	0.7902	0.8299	0.7935	0.8435

tion is included within it. Hence, we could potentially improve its performance by designing better neighborhood masks and by adding some shape information.

The segmentation results of two test cases are illustrated in Figs. 4 and 5. Figure 4 illustrates a relatively challenging case (Test case 5) which shows low similarity indices in the automatic segmentation. Not only does the patient have anabnormal

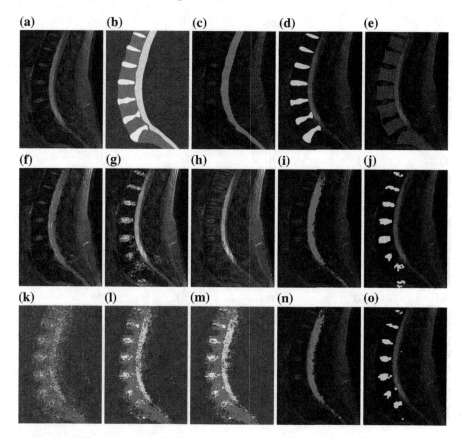

Fig. 4 Illustration of a challenging case showing low dice similarity indices (Test case 5): **a** shows the original mid-sagittal MRI, **b, c, d** and **e** show the manual segmentation (ground truth), **f, g** and **h** show the label maps for the dural sac, disc and vertebra respectively using Method 1, while **i** and **j** show the dural sac and disc segmentation after morphological post processing. **k, l** and **m** show the label maps generated at the end of iteration number 1, 6 and 200 respectively using Method 2 (Gibbs Sampling), while **n** and **o** show the dural sac and disc segmentation after morphological post processing

intervertebral disc (L5-S1), the intensity variations make automatic segmentation very difficult. Figure 5 illustrates another case (Test case 6) which shows good automatic segmentation results (high dice similarity indices) inspite of having an abnormal intervertebral disc (L5-S1).

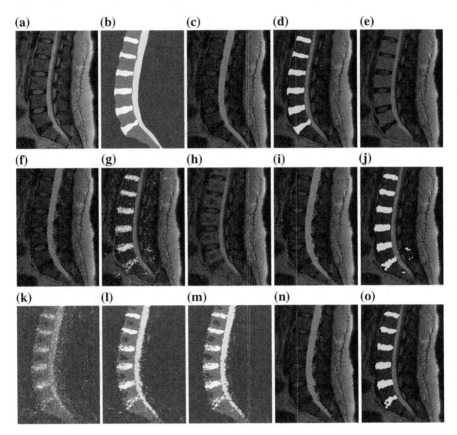

Fig. 5 Illustration of a case with high dice similarity indices (Test case 6): **a** shows the original mid-sagittal MRI, **b, c, d** and **e** show the manual segmentation (ground truth), **f, g** and **h** show the label maps for the dural sac, disc and vertebra respectively using Method 1, while **i** and **j** show the dural sac and disc segmentation after morphological post processing. **k, l** and **m** show the label maps generated at the end of iteration number 1, 6 and 200 respectively using Method 2 (Gibbs Sampling), while **n** and **o** show the dural sac and disc segmentation after morphological post processing

5 Conclusion and Future Work

We have proposed a supervised and unified approach towards complete segmentation of lumbar MRI. Using this approach we can simultaneously segment a sagittal slice into 4 class labels:dural sac, intervertebral disc, vertebra and background. We have also provided validation of our method using 53 clinical cases out of which 40 were used for training and the rest for testing. On an average, we achieved greater than 0.8 Dice Similarity Indices for both the dural sac and the intervertebral dics. Keeping in mind our encouraging results, we propose to experiment on larger datasets and also enhance our approach by incorporating shape and better neighborhood information into our model.

Acknowledgments This research was funded in part by NSF Grants DBI 0959870 and CNS 0855220 and NYSTAR grants 60701 and 41702.

References

1. Alomari, R.S., Corso, J.J., Chaudhary, V.: Labeling of lumbar discs using both pixel- and object-level features with a two-level probabilistic model. IEEE Trans. Med. Imaging **30**(1), 1–10 (2011)
2. Bhargavan, M., Sunshine, J.H., Schepps, B.: Too few radiologists? Am. J. Roentgenol. **178**(5), 1075–1082 (2002)
3. Bhole, C., Kompalli, S., Chaudhary, V.: Context-sensitive labeling of spinal structures in MRI images. In: The Proceedings of SPIE Medical Imaging (2009)
4. Breiman, L., Friedman, J., Olshen, R., Stone, C.: Classification Regression Trees. Wadsworth and Brooks, Monterey (1984)
5. Cherry, D.K., Hing, E., Woodwell, D.A., Rechtsteiner, E.A.: National ambulatory medical care survey: 2006 summary. Nati. Health Stat. Rep. **3**, 1–39 (2008)
6. Dalal, N., Triggs, B.: Histograms of oriented gradients for human detection. Int. Conf. Comput. Vis. Pattern Recogn. **2**, 886–893 (2005)
7. Ghosh, S., Alomari, R.S., Chaudhary, V., Dhillon, G.: Computer-aided diagnosis for lumbar mri using heterogeneous classifiers. In: Proceedings of the 8th IEEE International Symposium on Biomedical Imaging: From Nano to Macro, ISBI, pp. 1179–1182 (2011)
8. Ghosh, S., Malgireddy, M.R., Chaudhary, V., Dhillon, G.: A new approach to automatic disc localization in clinical lumbar MRI: Combining machine learning with heuristics. In: Proceedings of the 9th IEEE International Symposium on Biomedical Imaging: From Nano to Macro, ISBI, pp. 114–117 (2012)
9. Horsfield, M., Sala, S., Neema, M., Absinta, M., Bakshi, A., Sormani, M., Rocca, M., Bakshi, R., Filippi, M.: Rapid semi-automatic segmentation of the spinal cord from magnetic resonance images: Application in multiple sclerosis. Neuroimage (2010)
10. Koh, J., Kim, T., Chaudhary, V., Dhillon, G.: Automatic segmentation of the spinal cord and the dural sac in lumbar mr images using gradient vector flow field. In: Proceedings of the 32nd Annual International Conference of the IEEE Engineering in Medicine and Biology Society, EMBC, pp. 2117–2120 (2010)
11. Koh, J., Scott, P.D., Chaudhary, V., Dhillon, G.: An automatic segmentation method of the spinal canal from clinical mr images based on an attention model and an active contour model. In: Proceedings of the 8th IEEE International Symposium on Biomedical Imaging: From Nano to Macro, ISBI, pp. 1467–1471 (2011)
12. Kundel, H.L.: Measurement of observer agreement. In: RSNA, pp. 303–308 (2003)
13. Oktay, A.B., Akgul, Y.S.: Localization of the lumbar discs using machine learning and exact probabilistic inference. In: MICCAI (3) (2011)
14. Schmidt, S., Kappes, J., Bergtholdt, M., Pekar, V., Dries, S., Bystrov, D., Schnoerr, C.: Spine detection and labeling using a parts-based graphical model. In: Proceedings of the 20th International Conference on Information Processing in Medical Imaging, IPMI, vol. 4584, pp. 122–133 (2007)

Part V
Registration/Labeling

Automatic Segmentation and Discrimination of Connected Joint Bones from CT by Multi-atlas Registration

Tristan Whitmarsh, Graham M. Treece and Kenneth E. S. Poole

Abstract Many applications require the automatic identification of bone structures in CT scans. The segmentation of the bone at the joints, however, is a difficult task to automate since the separation of the bones can be reduced by a degradation of the articular cartilage. In addition, the bone boundary can become very thin at certain locations due to osteoporosis, making it difficult to discriminate between the bone and neighbouring soft tissue. In this work, therefore, a probabilistic method is proposed to segment the bone structures by the registration of multiple atlases. Several atlas combination strategies are evaluated with respect to the segmentation and discrimination of the proximal femur and pelvic bone, and the L2 and L3 vertebrae, on datasets of 30 subjects using a leave-one-out approach. The mean overlap is computed and a false overlap measure is proposed to assess the correct discrimination of the bone structures. In addition, the mean average surface distances and Hausdorff distances are computed on the surface meshes extracted from the label maps. The results indicate that a generalized local-weighted voting approach is preferred, which results in a mean overlap ≥ 0.97 for all bone structures, while being able to accurately discriminate between neighbouring bone structures.

T. Whitmarsh (✉) · G. M. Treece
Department of Engineering, University of Cambridge, Trumpington Street,
Cambridge CB2 1PZ, UK
e-mail: tw401@cam.ac.uk

G. M. Treece
e-mail: gmt11@eng.cam.ac.uk

K. E. S. Poole
Department of Medicine, Level 5, Addenbrooke's Hospital, University of Cambridge,
Box 157 , Hills Road, Cambridge CB2 2QQ, UK
e-mail: kp254@medschl.cam.ac.uk

J. Yao et al. (eds.), *Computational Methods and Clinical Applications*
for Spine Imaging, Lecture Notes in Computational Vision and Biomechanics 17,
DOI: 10.1007/978-3-319-07269-2_17, © Springer International Publishing Switzerland 2014

1 Introduction

Segmenting bone structures is of particular importance for orthopaedic surgical planning as well as implant selection and can aid in the diagnosis of pathologies such as osteoporosis, whereby the bone quality is examined, or osteoarthritis which requires an evaluation of the cartilage degradation.

Various bone segmentation methods have already been proposed with applications to segmenting the hip [1, 2], as well as the vertebrae [3, 4]. Segmenting joint bones, however, can become particularly difficult due to the thin cortex at certain regions which is exacerbated by osteoporosis. Moreover, the close proximity of the bone boundaries at the joints make it difficult to discriminate between adjacent bone structures. This in turn is aggravated by the presence of osteoarthritis, which reduces the cartilage and makes it difficult to determine where the bone ends and where the next begins. It therefore becomes necessary to include some form of *a priori* information into the bone segmentation method.

Statistical models have recently become popular in medical image segmentation and have already been applied to the segmentation of the proximal femur [5], the pelvic bone [6] and individual vertebrae [7]. These methods, however, often do not in a straightforward manner guarantee the separation of neighbouring bones. Moreover, the segmentation using statistical models is constrained to the main variations of the dataset used for training the model, thus not allowing the accurate segmentation of irregular pathological bones or outliers.

There has already been much research into segmenting brain structures in the field of neuroimaging where the connected brain tissue structures have to be identified and labelled to relate structural changes to neurological disorders. This is commonly done by the deformable registration of an atlas which is particularly suited to segmenting connected tissue structures as is the case with brain regions. Initially, a single-atlas registration was proposed and was later improved by the registration of multiple atlases [8], which can subsequently be merged through various combination strategies [9]. This was shown to result in segmentation accuracies exceeding all others and has rapidly become the standard in brain image segmentation.

Thus, in this work we apply the multi-atlas registration approach to the segmentation of connected joint bone structures and evaluate this technique for its ability to not only segment bone structures but also its ability to separate the connected bones. The method is evaluated for the hip whereby the proximal femur and hemipelvis are segmented and identified as well as the lumbar spine where the L2 and L3 vertebrae are individually labelled. The atlases are constructed by manual delineations of the bones and the segmentation method is evaluated in a leave-one-out analysis, giving the overlap measures and surface distances as the segmentation and discrimination accuracies.

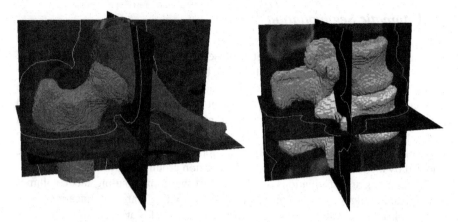

Fig. 1 Manual segmentations of the proximal femur and hemipelvis (*left*) and the vertebrae (*right*), shown here by the surfaces extracted from the labelled tissue regions within the volumes, with the region of interest for the registration process *outlined* in *white*

2 Materials and Methods

2.1 Data

A dataset of 30 CT scans of the pelvic area was collected which consists of only female subjects with an average age of 43.9 ± 14.8 years and ranging between 20 and 78 years.[1] A dataset of lumbar spine CT scans was also collected which consists of 9 male and 21 female subjects with a mean age of 57.6 ± 9.6 years and ranging between 12 and 71 years.[2] The pelvic CT scans were performed using the Siemens Sensation 64 Slice CT system (Siemens Healthcare, Erlangen, Germany) with a pixel spacing of 0.7×0.7 mm and slice spacing of 0.5 mm and the spinal scans using the GE LightSpeed 16 CT device (GE Healthcare, Madison, WI, USA) with a pixel spacing of 0.7×0.7 mm and slice spacing of 1.5 mm. All participants gave informed consent for the analysis of their hip, pelvic and vertebral imaging data.

For the pelvic volumes the right proximal femur was cropped below the lesser trochanter and the hemipelvis below the anterior superior iliac spine. Both the pelvic volumes and the spinal volumes were further cropped to contain only the bone structures of interest and the volumes were resampled to 1 mm cubic voxels. In the 30 pelvic CT scans the proximal femur and hemipelvis were manually labelled as well as the L2 and L3 vertebrae in the spinal CT scans. Thus, the atlases consist of the CT volumes with associated label maps, which delineate the bone regions (Fig. 1).

---

[1] MRC-Ageing: LREC 06/Q0108/180 study previously published in Poole et al., J Bone Miner Res, 2010.

[2] ACCT-1: LREC 04/Q0108/257 study previously published in McEniery et al., Hypertension, 2009.

2.2 Automatic Segmentation

For the automatic segmentation, the set of atlases are registered onto the target volume by means of an affine transformation followed by a multi-scale B-spline registration. For the multi-scale B-spline registration we used a control point spacing of 32, 16 and 8 mm consecutively whereby the displacement of the control points are constrained to 0.4 times the control point spacing to guarantee diffeomorphism [10]. The mutual information (MI) similarity measure was used for the registrations and a mask of the region of interest was defined by applying an appropriate threshold to the CT volume followed by a dilation to include a boundary region around the bone (Fig. 1).

The resulting transformations are applied to the corresponding label volumes using a nearest neighbour resampling, thereby propagating manual delineations from the multiple atlases to the target subject. Thus, for each of the atlases the voxels in the target volume are labelled as belonging to one of the bone structures or soft tissue.

Several common atlas combination strategies are evaluated to find one best suited for bone structures: a simple majority voting scheme, a global-weighted combination strategy, the statistical fusion method STAPLE [11] and generalized local-weighted voting. While majority voting assigns the tissue structure to each voxel based on the majority of the atlases, global weighted voting assigns a weight to each of the atlases based on the similarity between the registered atlas and the target volume. Here, the weights are determined by the mean squared error m within the region of interest, magnified by a gain p as m^p.

Generalized local-weighted voting computes the weights of the atlases at each voxel separately by taking the mean squared error in a cubic neighbourhood region of diameter d, which is again magnified by a gain p. Since local-weighted voting can result in irregular and disconnected bone structures when incorporating a relatively small region, in a post processing step a regularization is applied to the label map. For each voxel, if a majority of neighbouring voxels is assigned to a different tissue structure, the labelling is changed to this structure. A final multi-label connected component filter is applied to fill holes in the labelled regions and remove disconnected structures, which is also applied to the segmentations from the other combination strategies, although these generally do not result in such artefacts.

2.3 Evaluation

The segmentation accuracy is evaluated by a leave-one-out method whereby for each volume the remaining 29 atlases are used for the automatic segmentation, which is then compared to the manual segmentation. The various atlas combination strategies are evaluated, as well as the use of a single-atlas where each registered atlas is considered as an individual automatic segmentation.

As a measure for the segmentation accuracy the Mean Overlap (MO) is computed:

$$MO = \frac{2|A \cap B|}{|A| + |B|} \tag{1}$$

where A denotes the automatic segmentation and B the manual segmentation of the selected region. Although the Mean Overlap represents the segmentation accuracy of the individual bone structures, we are also interested in how well connected bones can be separated. Therefore, the overlap of the automatic segmentation with the manual segmentation of the neighbouring bone structure is computed as such:

$$\begin{aligned} FO_{femur-pelvis} &= \left|A_{femur} \cap B_{pelvis}\right| + \left|A_{pelvis} \cap B_{femur}\right| \\ FO_{L2-L3} &= |A_{L2} \cap B_{L3}| + |A_{L3} \cap B_{L2}| \end{aligned} \tag{2}$$

This False Overlap (FO) measure thus evaluates how well the two bones are discriminated from each other. A value of the gain for the global weighted voting is decided upon by examining the response of these measurements to a range of values for p. The accuracy of the local-weighted voting with respect to the MO and FO is assessed for a range of combinations of the diameter d of the cubical neighbourhood region and the gain p.

Finally, a surface mesh is extracted from the segmentations, which allows for the computation of the mean absolute Surface Distance (SD) as well as the Hausdorff distance (HD).

3 Results

For the global weighted voting a gain of $p = -2$ appeared to be a good compromise with respect to the MO and FO segmentation errors for the various bone structures and here this value is used for comparison with other combination strategies. In Table 1 the overlap measures and surface distances are given for all combination strategies. These results indicate that all multi-atlas strategies outperform the single-atlas segmentations method, while the generalized local-weighted voting combination strategy results in the best segmentation and discrimination for all measurements.

The bar graphs of Fig. 2 indicate that local-weighted voting using a single voxel is considerably less accurate with respect to the mean overlap of all bone structures and the FO between the vertebrae than incorporating a region with a diameter of 3 voxels, while using a greater region gradually decreases the segmentation and discrimination accuracy. A gain of $p = -1$ results in the best MO for the proximal femur and pelvis. However, although a gain of $p = -2$ results in a minimum decrease of the average MO, it results in a greatly reduced FO between the femur and pelvis. Furthermore, for the vertebrae a gain of $p = -2$ appears optimal. Thus, we propose the use of a 3 voxel diameter neighbourhood region with a gain of $p = -2$, which results in a MO of 0.988 ± 0.002 and 0.981 ± 0.005 for the proximal femur and hemipelvis respectively with a FO of 40.6 ± 48.1 and a MO of 0.967 ± 0.008 and 0.968 ± 0.007 for the L2 and L3 vertebrae with a FO between them of 40.2 ± 38.4.

Table 1 The Mean Overlap (MO), False Overlap (FO, mm³), mean absolute Surface Distance (SD, mm) and Hausdorff Distances (HD, mm) for several combination strategies and the single-atlas approach

		Single atlas	Majority voting	weighted voting	STAPLE	Local weighted voting
MO	Femur	0.970 ± 0.023	0.984 ± 0.004	0.985 ± 0.004	0.982 ± 0.005	0.988 ± 0.002
	Pelvis	0.958 ± 0.006	0.977 ± 0.004	0.978 ± 0.003	0.975 ± 0.005	0.981 ± 0.005
	L2	0.930 ± 0.010	0.960 ± 0.007	0.959 ± 0.007	0.955 ± 0.010	0.967 ± 0.008
	L3	0.929 ± 0.012	0.960 ± 0.007	0.960 ± 0.007	0.956 ± 0.010	0.968 ± 0.007
FO	Femur-Pelvis	161.9 ± 219.4	63.3 ± 50.1	62.9 ± 49.2	68.3 ± 55.4	40.6 ± 48.1
	L2-L3	178.7 ± 118.8	85.6 ± 64.4	82.2 ± 66.0	94.2 ± 60.4	40.2 ± 38.4
SD	Femur	0.49 ± 0.33	0.29 ± 0.07	0.28 ± 0.06	0.32 ± 0.09	0.23 ± 0.04
	Pelvis	0.46 ± 0.06	0.27 ± 0.04	0.27 ± 0.04	0.31 ± 0.06	0.24 ± 0.06
	L2	0.57 ± 0.07	0.36 ± 0.06	0.36 ± 0.06	0.40 ± 0.08	0.30 ± 0.07
	L3	0.59 ± 0.10	0.37 ± 0.05	0.37 ± 0.05	0.40 ± 0.08	0.30 ± 0.06
HD	Femur	4.83 ± 3.17	2.99 ± 2.07	2.85 ± 2.03	2.92 ± 2.10	2.98 ± 0.99
	Pelvis	6.02 ± 3.01	3.59 ± 2.33	3.58 ± 2.23	4.00 ± 2.71	2.98 ± 2.24
	L2	6.01 ± 2.05	3.60 ± 1.03	3.71 ± 1.04	3.78 ± 1.14	2.97 ± 0.95
	L3	6.48 ± 2.42	4.00 ± 1.22	3.93 ± 1.08	3.90 ± 1.32	3.06 ± 1.10

mean ± standard deviation

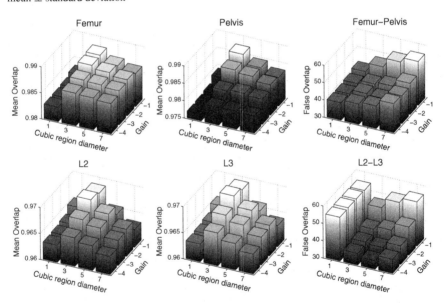

Fig. 2 The bar graphs of the Mean Overlap of the proximal femur and hemipelvis and False Overlap between the two for the various combinations of the cubical neighbourhood region diameter d and gain p (*top*) and the same measurements for the L2 and L3 vertebrae (*bottom*)

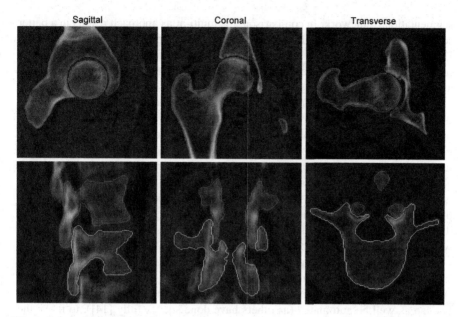

Fig. 3 Results of the automatic segmentations of the proximal femur and hemipelvis (*top*) and the individual vertebrae (*bottom*) using the proposed multi-atlas registration technique with the generalized local-weighted majority voting atlas combination strategy

In Fig. 3 the separation of the femoral head and the acetabulum are shown for one subject, as well as the critical regions of the vertebral segmentation of the articular processes as resulting from the local-weighted voting atlas combination strategy.

4 Discussion

In this work a multi-atlas based segmentation method for connected bone structures was proposed while evaluating the most common atlas combination strategies. In Table 1 we show that a local-weighted voting provides the best segmentation and discrimination accuracy for these selected bone structures, which is supported by Artaechevarria et al. [9] who state that a local method is preferred for high contrast regions, as is the case with bone contours.

Although the work of Hanaoka et al. [3] shows good results with respect to the vertebral bone segmentation with a mean surface error of 1.11 ± 0.40 mm and MO of 0.87 ± 0.04, this was improved by the use of a statistical model [7], which resulted in a mean surface error of 0.939 ± 0.410 mm and MO of 0.896 ± 0.046. A Hausdorff distance of 10.175 ± 3.184 mm was reported, which was ascribed to the errors at the processes. In [12] the lumbar vertebrae were segmented with a MO and Hausdorff distance of 0.893 ± 0.017 and 14.03 ± 1.40 mm respectively using a modified level set segmentation framework. In comparison, the multi-atlas approach results in a better segmentation accuracy for all combination strategies. In particular, the relatively low Hausdorff distances (2.97 ± 0.95 and 3.06 ± 1.10 mm for the L2 and L3 vertebrae respectively) indicate that the vertebral processes are also correctly segmented using a multi-atlas approach.

A mean surface distance for the pelvis and femur shapes of 1.20 mm was reported in [13] which incorporates a combined statistical model of the pelvis and proximal femur for the segmentation of diseased hips. In [5] a mean surface distance of 0.20 ± 0.063 mm and a MO of 0.992 ± 0.006 is reported for the segmentation of 10 proximal femurs using a shape-intensity prior model constructed from 12 CT scans. A similar, although slightly worse, surface error of 0.23 ± 0.04 mm and a MO of 0.988 ± 0.002 is achieved by the multi-atlas approach using generalized local-weighted voting. A direct comparison with previous work, however, is not appropriate due to the use of different populations with different levels of osteoporosis and cartilage reduction, as well as the use of a different evaluation method.

Although a localisation and initial alignment of the hip is straightforward, the identification of the individual vertebrae is not. In this work the CT volumes are cropped to contain the bones of interest resulting in an implicit initial alignment, but can as well be automated (as others have done successfully [14]), to make the process fully automatic.

The datasets used in this work consist of subjects with a wide range of ages of which some can be assumed to already have some bone and cartilage degradation. However, it does not specifically contain diseased bones. In particular osteoarthritis can cause the bones to be difficult to separate because of excessive cartilage reduction as well as unusual bone structures due to osteophytes. Considering that the method presented in this work is particularly suited for the segmentation of these bones, we aim to evaluate the multi-atlas segmentation method for these affected bones as well, once such a dataset becomes available to us.

To conclude, we have presented an automatic segmentation method which effectively segments and separates the individual bones within a complex joint structure, thereby potentially improving surgical planning and bone quality assessment with respect to diseases such as arthritis and osteoporosis.

Acknowledgments Tristan Whitmarsh receives research funding from Eli Lilly.

References

1. Zoroofi, R., Sato, Y., Sasama, T., Nishii, T., Sugano, N., Yonenobu, K., Yoshikawa, H., Ochi, T., Tamura, S.: IEEE Trans. Inf. Technol. Biomed. **7**(4), 329 (2003)
2. Krcah, M., Szekely, G., Blanc, R.: IEEE ISBI 2087–2090 (2011)
3. Hanaoka, S., Fritscher, K., Welk, M., Nemoto, M., Masutani, Y., Hayashi, N., K. Ohtomo, K., Schubert, R.: MICCAI, 554–561 (2011)
4. Ma, J., Lu, L., Zhan, Y., Zhou, X., Salganicoff, M., Krishnan, A.: MICCAI, 19–27 (2010)
5. Fritscher, K., Grünerbl, A., Schubert, R.: Int. J. CARS **1**(6), 341 (2007)

6. Seim, H., Kainmueller, D., Heller, M., Lamecker, H., Zachow, S., Hege, H.C.: EG VCBM, 93–100 (2008)
7. Hanaoka, S., Fritscher, K., Schuler, B., Masutani, Y., Hayashi, N., Ohtomo, K., Schubert, R.: SPIE Med. Imaging, **796**, 242–14 (2011)
8. Heckemann, R.A., Hajnal, J.V., Aljabar, P., Rueckert, D., Hammers, A.: Neuroimage **33**(1), 115 (2006)
9. Artaechevarria, X., Muñoz-Barrutia, A., de Solórzano, C.O.: IEEE Trans. Med. Imaging. **28**(8), 1266 (2009)
10. Rueckert, D., Aljabar, P., Heckemann, R., Hajnal, J., Hammers, A.: MICCAI, 702–709 (2006)
11. Warfield, S.K., Zou, K.H., Wells, W.M.: IEEE Trans. Med. Imaging **23**(7), 903 (2004)
12. Lim, P.H., Bagci, U., Bai, L.: IEEE Trans. Biomed. Eng. **60**(1), 115 (2013)
13. Yokota, F., Okada, T., Takao, M., Sugano, N., Tada, Y., Sato Y.: MICCAI, 811–818 (2009)
14. Glocker, B., Feulner, J., Criminisi, A., Haynor, D.R., Konukoglu, E.: MICCAI, 590–598 (2012)

Registration of MR to Percutaneous Ultrasound of the Spine for Image-Guided Surgery

Lars Eirik Bø, Rafael Palomar, Tormod Selbekk and Ingerid Reinertsen

Abstract One of the main limitations of today's navigation systems for spine surgery is that they often are not available until after the bone surface has been exposed. Also, they lack the capability of soft tissue imaging, both preoperatively and intraoperatively. The use of ultrasound has been proposed to overcome these limitations. By registering preoperative magnetic resonance (MR) images to intraoperative percutaneous ultrasound images, navigation can start even before incision. We therefore present a method for registration of MR images to ultrasound images of the spine. The method is feature-based and consists of two steps: segmentation of the bone surfaces from both the ultrasound images and the MR images, followed by rigid registration using a modified version of the Iterative Closest Point algorithm. The method was tested on data from a healthy volunteer, and the data set was successfully segmented and registered with an accuracy of 3.67 ± 0.38 mm.

L. E. Bø (✉) · T. Selbekk · I. Reinertsen
Department of Medical Technology, SINTEF Technology and Society, Trondheim, Norway
e-mail: lars.eirik.bo@sintef.no

T. Selbekk
e-mail: tormod.selbekk@sintef.no

I. Reinertsen
e-mail: ingerid.reinertsen@sintef.no

L. E. Bø · I. Reinertsen
Department of Circulation and Medical Imaging, Norwegian University of Science
and Technology, Trondheim, Norway

L. E. Bø
The Central Norway Regional Health Authority, Trondheim, Norway

R. Palomar
The Intervention Centre, Oslo University Hospital, Oslo, Norway
e-mail: rafael.palomar@rr-research.no

J. Yao et al. (eds.), *Computational Methods and Clinical Applications*
for Spine Imaging, Lecture Notes in Computational Vision and Biomechanics 17,
DOI: 10.1007/978-3-319-07269-2_18, © Springer International Publishing Switzerland 2014

1 Introduction

In spinal surgery today, many procedures are performed with no or only minimal image guidance. Preoperative computed tomography (CT) or magnetic resonance (MR) images are used for diagnosis and planning, but during surgery, two-dimensional C-arm fluoroscopy is widely used both for initial detection of the correct spinal level and for intra-operative imaging. Navigation systems exist, but mainly for placement of pedicle screws. These usually first come to use when the bone surface has been exposed. Using a simple landmark or surface registration method the preoperative CT image is then aligned with the patient and can be used for planning and guidance of the screws. A number of groups have evaluated the use of navigation for this purpose, and a review of the topic was presented by Tjardes et al. [12]. They conclude that the benefits of image-guidance in terms of accurate placement of the screws and reduced exposure to ionizing radiation have been proven, in particular for the cervical and lumbar procedures. In other areas of spine surgery, navigation and image guidance are still on the experimental stage.

One of the main limitations of today's navigation systems for spine surgery is that they often are not available until after the bone surface has been exposed. The use of ultrasound has been proposed to overcome this limitation. By registering preoperative images to intraoperative percutaneous ultrasound images, navigation can start before incision and therefore be used for both level detection and planning at an early stage of the procedure. Thus, the use of X-ray fluoroscopy can possibly be reduced.

In order to make a navigation system based on intraoperative ultrasound clinically useful, the greatest challenge is to achieve accurate and robust registration between the preoperative images and the ultrasound images with minimal user interaction. Registration of CT images of the spine to corresponding ultrasound images has been investigated by several groups, and two main approaches have been explored: feature-based registration and intensity-based registration. In the first case, corresponding features are extracted from the two datasets to be registered prior to registration. In the case of spine surgery, the feature of choice is the bone surface as this is the only feature that can be reliably detected in the ultrasound images. Segmentation of the bone surface from ultrasound images of the spine is still a challenging topic due to noise, artifacts and difficulties in imaging surfaces parallel to the ultrasound beam. A few methods have been described in the literature, ranging from simple ray tracing techniques [15] to more advanced methods based on probability measures [4, 7, 9] or phase symmetry [13]. Following surface extraction, the segmented bone surfaces are registered using the Iterative Closest Point (ICP) algorithm [2] or the unscented Kalman filter [9].

In intensity-based registration, a similarity metric based on the image intensities is optimized to find the spatial transformation that best maps one image onto the other [6, 8, 14, 15]. As MR/CT and ultrasound images present very different intensity and noise characteristics, a common approach is to create simulated ultrasound images from the pre-operative data and register the simulated image to the real ultrasound image. In these simulations, the direction of sound wave propagation, transmission, reflection and noise can be modelled in order to obtain images that can be reliably registered to real ultrasound images based on image intensities.

While these studies show a lot of promise, they focus almost exclusively on the registration of preoperative CT images. However, many spinal procedures, such as the treatment of disc herniations and intraspinal tumours, rely on the soft-tissue imaging capabilities of MR. Thus, by combining ultrasound imaging with preoperative MR, navigation could be extended to a variety of spinal procedures that do not benefit from image guidance today. In these procedures, the ultrasound could also be used for intraoperative imaging, reducing the use of fluoroscopy even further. As a first step towards this end, we present a method for registration of preoperative MR images to percutaneous ultrasound images of the spine, including a preliminary assessment of its performance.

2 Methods and Experiments

Our registration method is feature-based and consists of two steps: First, the bone surfaces are segmented from both the ultrasound images and the MR images, and then the two surfaces are registered using a modified version of the ICP algorithm.

2.1 Ultrasound Acquisition and Segmentation

The ultrasound images were acquired using a Vivid E9 scanner with an 11 MHz linear probe (GE Healthcare, Little Chalfont, UK). Some groups have used lower frequencies, which enable good imaging of deeper structures such as the transverse processes of the spine [6, 9, 13–15]. However, this makes imaging of superficial structures, such as the spinous processes and the sacrum, challenging. As these structures represent important features for the registration algorithm, we found that a relatively high frequency gave a better compromise between depth penetration and resolution. The ultrasound probe was tracked with the Polaris optical tracking system (NDI, Waterloo, ON, Canada), and both images and corresponding tracking data were recorded using the navigation system CustusX [1] with a digital interface to both the ultrasound scanner and the tracking system. The two-dimensional ultrasound images were also reconstructed to a three-dimensional volume using the Pixel Nearest Neighbor (PNN) reconstruction algorithm [11].

While the reconstructed, three-dimensional ultrasound volume is useful for navigation, the reconstruction process tends to introduce a certain blurring. The volume usually also has a lower resolution than the original, two-dimensional ultrasound images. We therefore used the latter as input to our segmentation method. In order to extract the bone surfaces from these images, we used a combination of the bone probability maps introduced by Jain et al. [7] and Foroughi et al. [4], and the backward scan line tracing presented by Yan et al. [15]. In ultrasound images, reflections from bone surfaces are seen as bright ridges perpendicular to the ultrasound beam. To calculate the probability of each pixel $a^{i,j}$ of the image A being part of such a ridge, the image was smoothed with a Gaussian filter, before calculating the Laplacian of Gaussian (LoG), i.e.

$$A_G = \{a_G^{i,j}\} = A * G \quad \text{and} \quad A_{LoG} = \{a_{LoG}^{i,j}\} = A_G * L, \tag{1}$$

where G and L are the convolution kernels of the Gaussian filter and the LoG filter respectively. This is a common operation in blob detection and usually produces a strong positive response for dark blobs and a strong negative response for bright blobs. To enhance the bright reflections, the positive values were therefore set to zero before taking the absolute value of the rest. The result was then added to the smoothed version of the original image to produce an initial bone probability map $P_1 = \{p_1^{i,j}\}$, i.e.

$$p_1^{i,j} = a_G^{i,j} + |\max\{a_{LoG}^{i,j}, 0\}|. \tag{2}$$

The other feature to be considered was the intensity profile in the propagation direction of the ultrasound. For a bone surface, this is typically characterized by a sudden, sharp peak followed by a dark shadow. To calculate the probability of a given pixel representing the maximum of such a profile, each scan line was considered separately. Assuming p_1^m is the mth pixel of the initial bone probability map P_1 along a given scan line, the secondary bone probability of this pixel was found as

$$p_2^m = p_1^m - \frac{p_1^{m-\delta} + p_1^{m+\delta}}{2} - \frac{\omega}{\lambda} \sum_{n=1}^{\lambda} p_1^{m+\delta+n}, \tag{3}$$

where 2δ is the width of a typical intensity peak and λ is the length of a typical bone shadow, both given in pixels. In our case, these were set to $\delta = 24$ and $\lambda = 322$, which corresponds to 1.5 and 20 mm respectively. ω is a weight that can be adjusted according to the overall noise level of the bone shadows in the image, and in our case this was set to 10.

The first term in (3) is simply the intensity of the mth pixel. At a bone reflection, this will be high and lead to a high bone probability. The second term combines the intensities at the distance δ behind and in front of the mth pixel. At a sharp peak of width 2δ, both of these will be low and have little impact on the bone probability. On the other hand, if there is no such peak, at least one of these will be high and lead to a reduced bone probability. The last term is the average intensity of the pixels in the shadow region behind the peak. If there is a lot of signal in this area, this term will be high and thus reducing the bone probability

Finally, we applied a variant of the backward scan line tracing to the resulting probability map: For each scan line, starting at the bottom of the image, the first local maximum above a certain threshold was deemed part of a bone surface. This was

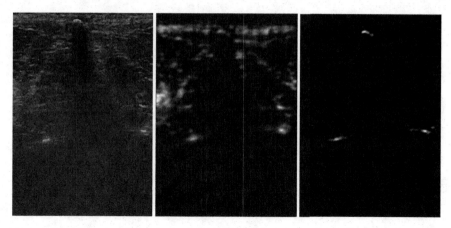

Fig. 1 An ultrasound image of a vertebra with the segmentation overlaid in *red* (*left*), the initial bone probability map (*centre*) and the final bone probability map after applying the threshold (*right*) (see colour figure online)

repeated for all the recorded images, and based on the corresponding tracking data, all points were transformed into the three-dimensional reference space of the tracking system. A typical example of both the probability maps and the final segmentation of an image is shown in Fig. 1. The method was implemented in MATLAB (MathWorks, Natick, MA, USA).

2.2 MR Acquisition and Segmentation

The MR images were acquired using an Achieva 3.0 T scanner (Philips Healthcare, Amsterdam, Netherlands). In order to facilitate both the segmentation of the spine and the subsequent navigation, we customized a full, three-dimensional MR protocol which enhanced the contrast between the bone and the surrounding soft tissue. This had a field of view of $80 \times 560 \times 560$ voxels and a voxel size of $1 \times 0.48 \times 0.48$ mm^3. The lumbar vertebrae were segmented using a semiautomatic method based on active contours implemented in the segmentation software ITK-SNAP [16]. However, in the area of the sacrum, the contrast between the bone and the surrounding soft tissue was lower, and here active contours driven by robust statistics resulted in more accurate segmentations. For this part, we therefore employed the Robust Statistics Segmentation (RSS) module [5] included in the medical imaging analysis and visualization software 3D Slicer [3].

The use of active contours for segmentation may lead to oversegmentation of certain anatomical structures, known as leaks. In MR images, such leaks are especially prominent in areas with motion artifacts caused by the patient not lying completely still during the image acquisition. This is often a problem, especially for patients in

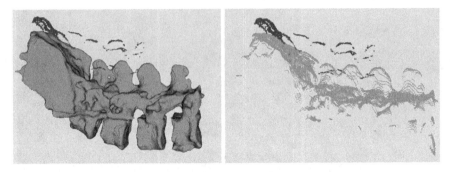

Fig. 2 The segmented ultrasound (*blue*) and MR (*red*) surfaces (*left*) and the same surfaces after reducing the MR surface with ray tracing (*right*) (see colour figure online)

need of spine surgery. To compensate for this, minor corrections of the segmentation results were performed manually for both the lumbar area and the sacrum.

The surface segmented from the MR volume represented the entire lumbar spine, and consisted therefore of a large number of points. However, only the surfaces facing the ultrasound probe were visible in the ultrasound images. Thus, a significant portion of the surface points in the segmented MR were irrelevant to the registration, as there were no corresponding points in the ultrasound images. To reduce the amount of data, and thus the work load of the registration algorithm, we therefore used a simple ray tracing method (posterior to anterior) to extract those points that were facing the ultrasound probe. An example of the resulting reduced surface can be seen in Fig. 2.

2.3 Registration

Following segmentation, the segmented surfaces from ultrasound and MR were imported into the navigation system for registration. Like all automatic registration methods, the ICP algorithm requires an initialization or a reasonable starting point in order to converge to the correct solution. This was provided by assuming that the two volumes covered approximately the same volume, that the first recorded ultrasound image was positioned at the sacrum and that the probe trajectory was from the sacrum upwards. The two image volumes were then aligned by first rotating the MR volume in order to align the x, y and z axes in the two volumes, and then translating the MR volume in order to align the points corresponding to the voxels $(n_x/2, 0, 0)$ in both volumes, where n_x is the number of voxels in the x-direction (patient left-to-right).

After this initial alignment, we used the ICP algorithm to rigidly register the reduced MR surface to the ultrasound surface. In order to reduce the influence of possible outliers on the registration result, the algorithm was modified by incorporating the Least Trimmed Squares (LTS) robust estimator as described by Reinertsen et al. [10].

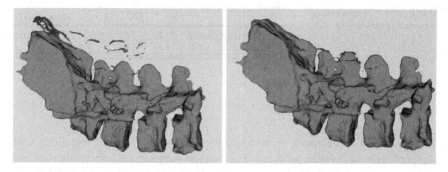

Fig. 3 The ultrasound (*blue*) and MR (*red*) surfaces after the initial alignment (*left*) and after the final registration (*right*) (see colour figure online)

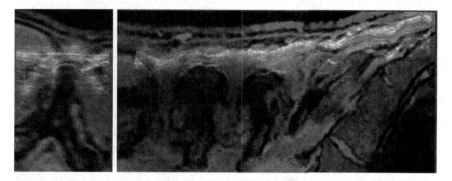

Fig. 4 A transverse slice (*left*) and a sagittal slice (*right*) from the ultrasound volume overlaid on *top* of the corresponding slices from the registered MR volume. The ultrasound data is shown in *red* and *yellow* and the MR data is shown in *grey* tones (see colour figure online)

2.4 Experiments

In order to evaluate our method, we acquired both ultrasound and MR images of the spine of a healthy volunteer. The only structures that were clearly discernible in both of these images were the top points of the spinous processes of three lowest vertebrae (L3, L4 and L5). These were therefore selected as control points and manually identified in both the original ultrasound volume and the MR volume. The surfaces were then registered to each other using the method described above, and the distances between the landmarks both after initial alignment and after final registration were computed.

Table 1 Distance between the control points in mm

	L3	L4	L5	Mean ± STD
After initial alignment	23.29	21.27	22.40	22.32 ± 1.01
After final registration	3.86	3.93	3.23	3.67 ± 0.38

3 Results

Through careful optimization of the acquisition protocols, both MR and ultrasound images of high quality were achieved. The data sets were successfully segmented and registered using the methods described above. Figure 3 shows the extracted surfaces both after the initial alignment and after rigid registration. The match can also be seen in Fig. 4, which shows transverse and sagittal views of corresponding ultrasound and MR volumes after registration. Finally, the distances between the control points before and after registration are given in Table 1.

4 Discussion

We have demonstrated that registration between MR and ultrasound images is feasible. The accuracy of 3.67 ± 0.38 mm is clinically relevant as it is sufficient to ensure that we are on the correct level. It is also comparable to that of many of the studies mentioned in the introduction. Still, this is a work in progress, and the results shown here are only preliminary.

It has been pointed out that intensity-based registration has an advantage over feature-based methods in that it makes use of all the information in the image, rather than just that of the bone surfaces [6]. In the case of spine imaging, however, other structures that are visible in the ultrasound images, such as muscle fibres and fat layers, are not imaged very well by neither CT nor MR. Their contribution to the registration procedure is therefore questionable.

The ultrasound images that we have acquired vary considerably in appearance from subject to subject. At the moment, this means that the parameters of the segmentation method, such as the width δ of the reflections, the length λ of the shadows and the weight ω must be manually adjusted to the particular data set. In the future, these adjustment should be done automatically, e.g. based on overall image statistics.

The MR segmentation methods that we presented here are only semiautomatic and quite time consuming. However, the result of this was a complete segmentation of the lumbar spine, and as we have already pointed out, only a small part of this information was actually relevant to the registration. We are therefore investigating methods to segment only the part of the anatomy that is most critical to the registration, i.e. the sacrum and the spinous and transverse processes. The results are promising, and it should be possible to perform this segmentation both quickly and with minimal user interaction.

The last component of the method is the registration. Here, we have shown that a reasonable rigid registration can be achieved using the ICP algorithm. However, the spine is flexible, and the change in curvature from the MR scanner, where the patient is lying in a supine position, to the operating room, where the patient is placed in a prone position, can be large. A group-wise rigid registration method, like the one proposed e.g. by Gill et al. [6] where only the space between the vertebrae is deformed, would be more appropriate.

Finally, our method needs more extensive testing, both with respect to robustness to anatomical variations and with respect to accuracy. The distance measure that we have used here, based on manual identification of landmarks, gives a good indication of the registration accuracy, but we should include a measure of inter- and intra-observer variability. Such measures could therefore be complimented with other assessment methods, such as phantom studies where the exact geometry is known and a reliable ground truth thus can be established. All of the above are currently addressed in our research.

5 Conclusion

The presented method is capable of registering MR images to percutaneous ultra-sound images of the spine. The registration accuracy is clinically relevant, and with minor improvements the user interaction can be reduced to a minimum. This method is thus an important step towards the realisation of a system for MR- and ultrasound-guided spine surgery.

Acknowledgments The work was funded through the user-driven research-based innovation project VIRTUS (The Research Council of Norway Grant No. 219326, SonoWand AS) and through a PhD grant from the Liaison Committee between the Central Norway Regional Health Authority (RHA) and the Norwegian University of Science and Technology.

References

1. Askeland, C., et al.: CustusX: A Research application for image-guided therapy. MIDAS J. 1–8 (2011). Systems and Architectures for Computer Assisted Interventions 2011. http://www.midasjournal.org/browse/journal/60
2. Besl, P.J., et al.: A method for registration of 3-D shapes. IEEE Trans. Pattern Anal. Mach. Intell. **14**(2), 239–256 (1992)
3. Fedorov, A., et al.: 3D slicer as an image computing platform for the quantitative imaging network. Magn. Reson. Imaging **30**(9), 1323–1341 (2012)
4. Foroughi, P., et al.: Ultrasound bone segmentation using dynamic programming. In: Yuhas, M.P. (ed.) IEEE ultrasonics symposium on 2007, pp. 2523–2526 (2007)
5. Gao, Y., et al.: A 3D interactive multi-object segmentation tool using local robust statistics driven active contours. Med. Image Anal. **16**(6), 1216–1227 (2012)
6. Gill, S., et al.: Biomechanically constrained groupwise ultrasound to CT registration of the lumbar spine. Med. Image Anal. **16**(3), 662–674 (2012)

7. Jain, A.K., et al.: Understanding bone responses in B-mode ultrasound images and automatic bone surface extraction using a bayesian probabilistic framework. In: Walker, W.F., Emelianov, S.Y. (eds.) Medical Imaging 2004: Ultrasonic Imaging and Signal Processing, Proceedings of SPIE, vol. 5373, pp. 131–14 (2004)

8. Lang, A., et al.: Multi-modal registration of speckle-tracked freehand 3D ultrasound to CT in the lumbar spine. Med. Image Anal. **16**(3), 675–686 (2012)

9. Rasoulian, A., et al.: Feature-based multibody rigid registration of CT and ultrasound images of lumbar spine. Med. Phys. **39**(6), 3154–3166 (2012)

10. Reinertsen, I., et al.: Validation of vessel-based registration for correction of brain shift. Med. Image Anal. **11**(4), 374–388 (2007)

11. Solberg, O.V., et al.: 3D ultrasound reconstruction algorithms from analog and digital data. Ultrasonics **51**(4), 405–419 (2011)

12. Tjardes, T., et al.: Image-guided spine surgery: state of the art and future directions. Eur Spine J **19**(1), 25–45 (2010)

13. Tran, D., et al.: Automatic Detection of Lumbar Anatomy in Ultrasound Images of Human Subjects. IEEE Trans Biomed Eng **57**(9), 2248–2256 (2010)

14. Winter, S., et al.: Registration of CT and intraoperative 3-D ultrasound images of the spine using evolutionary and gradient-based methods. IEEE Trans. Evol. Comput. **12**(3), 284–296 (2008)

15. Yan, C.X.B., et al.: Ultrasound-CT registration of vertebrae without reconstruction. Int. J. Comput. Assist. Radiol. Surg. **7**(6), 901–909 (2012)

16. Yushkevich, P.A., et al.: User-guided 3D active contour segmentation of anatomical structures: significantly improved efficiency and reliability. NeuroImage **31**(3), 1116–1128 (2006)

Vertebrae Detection and Labelling in Lumbar MR Images

Meelis Lootus, Timor Kadir and Andrew Zisserman

Abstract We describe a method to automatically detect and label the vertebrae in human lumbar spine MRI scans. The method is based on detections in all slices of sagittal MRI scans of arbitrary slice spacing. Our contribution is to show that marrying two strong algorithms (the DPM object detector of Felzenszwalb et al. [1], and inference using dynamic programming on chains) together with appropriate modelling, results in a simple, computationally cheap procedure, that achieves state-of-the-art performance. The training of the algorithm is principled, and heuristics are not required. The method is evaluated quantitatively on a dataset of 371 MRI scans, and it is shown that the method copes with pathologies such as scoliosis, joined vertebrae, deformed vertebrae and disks, and imaging artifacts. We also demonstrate that the same method is applicable (without retraining) to CT scans.

1 Introduction

The task dealt with in this paper is the following: given an MR scan of the lumbar spine, localize and label all the vertebrae present in that image. The motivation for this work is that spine appearance, shape and geometry measurements are necessary

Funded by ESPRC.
Financial support was provided by ERC grant VisRec no. 228180.

M. Lootus (✉) · T. Kadir · A. Zisserman
Engineering Science Department, Oxford University, Parks Road, Oxford, UK
e-mail: meelis@robots.ox.ac.uk

T. Kadir
e-mail: timork@mirada-medical.co.uk

A. Zisserman
e-mail: az@robots.ox.ac.uk

J. Yao et al. (eds.), *Computational Methods and Clinical Applications*
for Spine Imaging, Lecture Notes in Computational Vision and Biomechanics 17,
DOI: 10.1007/978-3-319-07269-2_19, © Springer International Publishing Switzerland 2014

Input   Output

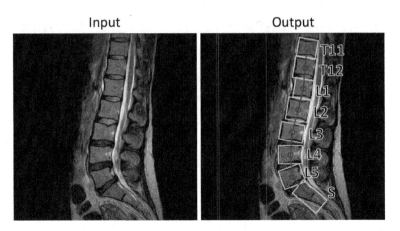

Fig. 1 The task. Given a 3D MR lumbar spine image comprising of a stack of sagittal 2D slices as input (the mid-slice is shown on the *left*), localize and label in that 3D image all the vertebrae that are present. The output (projected on the mid-slice on the *right*) consists of labelled tight bounding boxes around the vertebrae. *Note* that all the 2D slices in the 3D slice stack are searched for vertebrae candidates

for abnormality detection *locally* at each disk [2–7] and vertebrae [8, 9] (such as herniation), as well as *globally* for the whole spine (such as spinal scoliosis).

In more detail, the input 3D image is a (sparsely spaced) stack of 2D sagittal images, and the output consists of labelled tight bounding boxes with labels around all the vertebrae in the image. Each bounding box is specified by its position, orientation, and scale. An example of the detection and labelling for a typical normal scan is shown in Fig. 1.

This detection task is challenging for a number of reasons, including: (1) the repetitive nature of the vertebrae, (2) varying image resolution and imaging protocols; artefacts, and (3) large anatomical and pathological variation, particularly in the lumbar spine. Various examples of challenging cases in our dataset are highlighted in Fig. 2. The anatomy and pathology variation can affect both the local vertebrae / disks appearance (e.g. degraded disks—Fig. 2h), and the global layout of the spine (e.g. scoliosis—Fig. 2c).

Contributions. Our method brings together two strong algorithms—the Deformable Part Model of Felzenszwalb et al. [1] based on Histogram of Oriented Gradients (HOG) image descriptors [10] and efficient inference on graphical models [11, 12]— making the algorithm accurate, robust, and efficient on challenging spine datasets. The algorithm is also tolerant to varying MR acquisition protocols, image resolutions, patient position, and varying slice spacing unlike related solutions in the literature. It localizes all the vertebrae present in a scan, and labels them correctly as long as the sacrum is present in the scan. Importantly, the method is appliccable to standard MRI protocols.

The method has two distinct stages. First, vertebrae candidates are detected by using a sliding window detector searching over position, scale, and angle (Sect. 2.1).

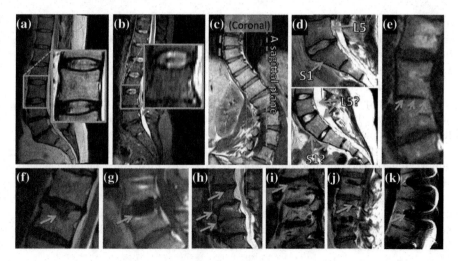

Fig. 2 Spine variation in our data. A collection of example images showing assorted image, anatomical and pathological modes of global variation of the spine shape, and local variation of the vertebrae, and the disks. Our algorithm is robust to all those variations. Abnormalities have been highlighted by the *red arrows*. **a** Normal spine with a zoom on a normal vertebra. **b** A low-resolution image. **c** A coronal view of a scoliotic spine, resulting in the spine not being cut by a single sagittal slice. **d** *Top* a normal sacrum, with unambiguous L5, S1 labelling based on shape and S1 and L5 orientation. *Bottom* a sacrum with ambiguous L5, S1 labelling based on their shape and orientation. **e** Joined vertebrae. **f–j** Pathologically deformed vertebrae and disks. **k** Magnetic susceptibility imaging artefacts

Second, a graphical model is fitted to the set of candidate detections to find the optimal spine layout and labelling based on the unary SVM score of the detection for each part, and a spatial cost between each pair of connected parts (Sect. 2.2). The HOG descriptor captures the near rectangular shape of the vertebrae. We detect vertebrae rather than disks since the vertebrae shape is more consistent than the disk shape as the lumbar spine studies are more often aimed at targeting disk deformations, and more suitable to be modelled with HOG. Disk locations can easily be found after detecting vertebrae.

The closest previous work to ours is that of Oktay and Akgul [13]. They detect disks and vertebrae in the lumbar spine using a Pyramid HOG descriptor; however, they only detect six disks and vertebrae with their graphical model, require the existence of both T1 and T2 scans to first detect the spinal cord, and they have a separate HOG template for each vertebra. In contrast, we demonstrate that just one generic vertebrae detector suffices for all vertebrae, and only require the T2 scan. Furthermore, they only use the mid-sagittal slices, making it only applicable to cases where all the spine parts are in the mid-sagittal slice, whereas we sequentially search for vertebrae in all the 2D images in the 3D stack (not restricted to the mid-sagittal slice).

Ghosh et al. [14] also use HOG features [10], however they do not label the vertebrae and make strong use of heuristics and information from complementary axial scans. They detect disks rather than vertebrae. Zhan et al. [15] present a robust hierarchical algorithm to detect and label arbitrary numbers of vertebrae and disks in nearly arbitrary field of view scans, as long as one of four 'anchor' vertebrae (C2, T1, L1, S) are present. They first detect the 'anchor' vertebrae, and then other 'bundle' vertebrae connected to it graphically. Although the method works very well within its domain, it requires isotropic 2.1 mm resolution scans which limits its applicability severely. Our method is not limited to this domain and, in particular, does not require the high isotropic resolution.

A further extensive body of literature on spine localization and labelling exists. In almost all the papers, the algorithms work in two stages. First, some anatomical parts characteristic of the spine are detected (vertebrae [16–18]/disks [14, 19–21]/both [13, 15]). Second, a spine layout model is fitted to the candidates to determine the best hypothesis for the spine layout. The spatial configuration of the spine parts, and in some cases also their individual characteristics [15, 18, 22], are taken into account to both label the disks and/or vertebra, and localize the spine.

2 Method

We present a method to localize and label vertebrae in lumbar MR images using two HOG-based detectors and a graphical model. First, given a stack of sagittal MR slices, vertebrae and sacrum candidates are detected using latent SVM on HOG in each slice as described in Sect. 2.1. Next, after local non-maxima suppression, the vertebrae candidates corresponding to the spine are picked and labelled by fitting a graphical model, as explained in Sect. 2.2.

2.1 Spine Part Detection

The spine part (vertebrae) detection is implemented using two detectors constituting latents SVMs on Histogram of Oriented Gradients (HOG) descriptors [10] using the Felzenszwalb VOC Challenge object detection framework [23]. We learn one generic 2D detector for vertebrae bodies (VBs), trained on all VBs in all the training images, and another more specific 2D detector for the sacrum, trained on the VBs of the first two links of the sacrum. Both the models are visualized along with a set of training samples in Fig. 3.

Training. Both the generic vertebrae body (VB) detector and the sacrum detector are trained using the Felzenszwalb detection framework [23]. The positive training examples for the VB detector are tight bounding boxes around the vertebral bodies of T10...L5 vertebrae with the bounding box sides parallel to the vertebral facets as shown in Fig. 3a. The positive training examples for the sacrum detector are tight bounding boxes around the first two links of the sacrum, with one side parallel to the posterior side of the sacrum as shown in Fig. 3b. The bounding boxes for both the VB

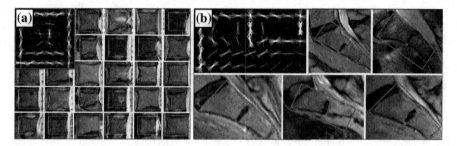

Fig. 3 The appearance model. Some training examples and a learned HOG template are shown for both the generic vertebrae body detector (**a**) and for the sacrum detector (**b**). The examples have been hand-annotated with tight Ground Truth bounding boxes as shown above and explained in Fig. 5

and the sacrum are defined by fitting a minimum bounding rectangle to landmarks on them—four for the VB and eight for the sacrum. Each training sample is extracted from the slice cutting through the middle of the respective vertebral body.

For the VB detector, four HOG templates are trained, each of them of a different aspect ratio. The HOG templates are each 6 cells high, and 6, 7, 8, and 9 cells wide, corresponding to aspect ratios between 1 and 1.5. The HOG cell size for the VB model is 8×8 pixels. The HOG template for the sacrum detector is 9 cells high by 5 cells wide, with 8×8 pixel HOG cell size. The HOG feature vectors are 31-dimensional, with 18 contrast-sensitive, 9 contrast-insensitive direction bins; and 4 texture feature bins.

The HOG templates capture the rectangular shape of the vertebrae, with variations due to deformation, and the trapezoid shape of the first two links of the sacrum. The vertebrae show wide size and resolution variation and are all scaled and warped to match one of the aspect ratios at training. The model is learned iteratively in several steps, with new positive samples mined by running the detector on the positive samples, collecting the strongest detections as new positives, and training a new detector using the new positives.

The negative samples for the vertebrae detector are first picked randomly from mid-slices with a hand-drawn black polygon covering all the vertebral bodies. Next, an iterative learning procedure is employed to pick hard negatives as false positive detections on the negative training images as detailed in [23].

Testing. During the candidate detection step at test time, a previously unseen sagittal scan is taken as input, and tight bounding boxes around vertebrae candidates are returned as output. The candidate search is performed sequentially in all slices of the scan. The VB and sacrum detector are run on each slice of the scan, searching over position, scale, and angle, with the scan rotated by $-20°$ to $20°$ in $10°$ increments. A feature pyramid is calculated for each angle, with HOG cells placed densely next to each other. The feature pyramid has 10 levels per doubling of resolution (10 levels per octave), with the image resized and resampled to $2\times$ the original size to $0.5\times$ the original size from the finest to coarsest scale. All the detections at all positions, scales,

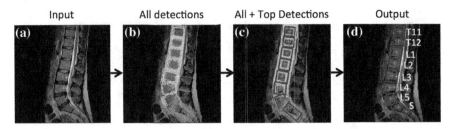

Fig. 4 Vertebrae detection pipeline. **a** Input image. **b** All detections at all rotation angles and scales. The *green rectangles* are generic vertebrae, and the *red rectangles* are sacrum candidates. **c** All detections, with top detections shown in thick *blue line*, and the "+" mark the ground truth vertebrae center locations. **d** Output detection bounding boxes along with the ground truths and labels

orientations are collected and transformed onto the original test image coordinate system as shown in Fig. 4.

A greedy non-maxima suppression algorithm is employed to remove most of the false positive detections in each slice as follows. First, the top-scoring bounding box is retained, and all bounding boxes overlapping it more than 50 % are discarded. Next, the second-highest scoring remaining bounding box is retained, and the discarding and retention process continues until all the remaining bounding boxes have at most 50 % overlap.

Next, the remaining bounding boxes from all the slices are collected and projected onto a single slice, and the non-maxima suppression process is repeated to end up with bounding boxes across all the slices that have at most 50 % overlap. These bounding boxes are next passed as input to the Graphical Model as described in Sect. 2.2 in order to eliminate any remaining false positives, and to label the vertebrae.

2.2 Graphical Model for Spine Layout

We train a parts-based graphical model [12] connecting the vertebrae in a chain. The graphical model takes as input the detections after non-maxima suppression described in the previous subsection, and gives as output the placement and labels of all vertebrae in the image. The method deals with multiple slices by ignoring the slice index in inference. The spine layout is given as a configuration $L = (l_1, l_2, \ldots, l_{n-1}, l_n)$ where l_i are the vertebra locations, with l_1 the C1 and $l_n = l_{25}$ the sacrum. The optimal configuration L^* of the graphical model is

$$L^* = \arg\min_L \left(\sum_{i=1}^n m_i\,(l_i) + \sum_{v_{i,j} \in G} d_{ij}\,(l_i, l_j) \right) \quad (1)$$

where l_i and l_j denote the vertebrae locations $l = (x_i, y_i, height_i, width_i, \theta_i)$ given by their location (x, y), size $(height, width)$, and orientation θ_i. The best model fit minimizes the sum of the unary appearance mismatch terms m_i from the part detectors output and the spatial deformation cost d_{ij} for connected pairs ij of parts, laid at l_i and l_j respectively. The last appearance term value m_{25} comes from the sacrum detector, and the rest of the appearance term values come from the universal vertebra detector. The spatial deformation cost is a sum of box functions on x and y coordinates, the ratio of vertebrae areas A_i & A_j, and the angle between the vertebrae:

$$d_{ij}(l_i, l_j) = S(A_i/A_j) + T(x_i - x_j) + U(y_i - y_j) + V(\theta_i - \theta_j) \qquad (2)$$

Here S, T, U, and V are the box functions on area A, position x & y, and angle θ that take a low constant value if their arguments are within favourable range of each other and a higher constant value if their arguments are outside that range.

To speed up the fitting process, a Viterbi message passing scheme from [12] for fast inference in $O(nh^2)$ time is employed where n is the number of parts and h the number of candidates per part. Typically, there are around $h = 100$ candidate positions per part, and the full inference takes around 0.1 s per MR volume. The full detection process from input to output typically takes less than a minute.

Training. The edges for the box functions S, T, U, and V are found as the minimum and maximum argument values of those functions on the training set (e.g. the minimum and maximum x-distance between L1 and L2 for T, etc.).

Testing. At test time, the whole model is fitted to the retained states, with extra "hidden" states with outside-FOV position for each part, with a penalty value for the "hidden" state learnt at training time [24]. At each position in the scan, the highest-scoring detection across all slices is retained for graphical model fitting as explained in Sect. 2.1. All retained states can be in different slices.

3 Experiments

3.1 Data, Annotation and Evaluation

The dataset consists of 371 MRI T2-weighted lumbar scans, acquired under various protocols. The scans contain normal and various abnormal cases as illustrated in Fig. 2. The dataset is split into 80 training and 291 testing images. The scans have isotropic in-slice resolution varying from 0.34 to 1.64 mm with mean at 0.78, median at 0.84 mm; and varying slice spacing from 3 to 5 mm, with 4 mm in almost all scans. The scans range in fields of view, containing 7–23 vertebrae starting from the sacrum, with median at 10 per scan.

Annotation. The scans were hand-annotated with two types of ground truth as illustrated in Fig. 5: (i) All the vertebrae centres in all the scans are marked with a point ("+" in Fig. 5), and labelled with the vertebrae name; and (ii) all the training scans

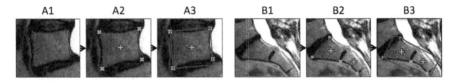

Fig. 5 The ground truth annotation process. A1-A3 show the generic vertebral, and B1-B3 the sacrum annotation process. There are two types of annotation: single point (the *green* "+" in the figure—used for testing) and bounding box (the *red rectangle*—used for training). Given an input (A1, B1), the points ("+" and "×") are hand-placed (A2,B2). The bounding box annotation is found as the minimal bounding rectangle to the "×" points around the vertebra/sacrum boundary. There are four boundary points for vertebrae (**a**) and eight for the sacrum (**b**)

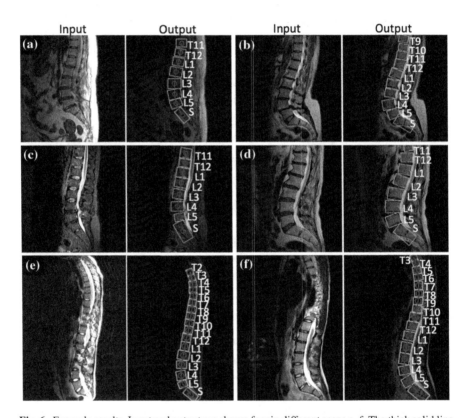

Fig. 6 Example results. Input and output are shown for six different scans a–f. The thick solid line rectangles show the detections for each vertebrae, along with their anatomical labels. *Note* how the algorithm is robust to varying field of view, resolution, and anatomy. *Note* that for visualization purposes, only mid-sagittal slices are shown and all the bounding boxes projected on them, however all the slices are searched for vertebrae candidates and the highest scoring ones retained

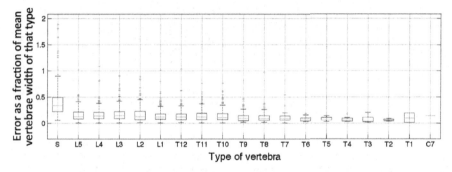

Fig. 7 Localization error by vertebrae type. Boxplots representing detection errors are shown. The error for a given vertebra type is calculated as the distance between the center of the detected bounding box and the ground truth vertebra center, divided by the mean width of that vertebra. The mean vertebrae widths are evaluated based on the bounding boxes on the training set. The horizontal line in the middle of each box is the median error, and the bottom and top of each box are the 25 and 75 percentile errors respectively. The bottom and top error bar end are the 5 and 95 percentile errors respectively, and the '+' denote statistical outliers

plus some test scans are annotated with a tight bounding box around each vertebra (Fig. 5A3, B3). The tight bounding boxes were defined by points ("×" in Fig. 5) along the vertebrae boundaries as shown.

Evaluation protocol. The detections are evaluated against vertebrae-center and the sacrum-center ground truth points. A positive detection for the sacrum is counted if a detected sacrum bounding box contains the sacrum ground truth point and does not contain any vertebrae center ground truth points. A positive detection for the vertebrae is counted if a detected vertebra bounding box contains one and only one ground truth point for a vertebral body, including the sacrum. This evaluation protocol ensures that the cases where a detection is much larger than the vertebral body, covering several vertebrae, are not counted as positive.

3.2 Results

The algorithm is evaluated on a set of 291 lumbar spine test images with variable number of vertebrae visible. Given an input scan, both the sacrum and vertebrae detectors are run on the scan, searching over position, scale, and angle. The position search is dense, the scale varies from 0.25 to 2 of the original image size (scale = 1) in small increments (so that there are 10 different scales per doubling of image size). The angle search runs from $-20°$ to $20°$ for vertebrae and $-60°$ to $0°$ for the sacrum in $10°$ increments.

Example outputs are shown in Fig. 6, and statistical results on localization error over the test set are plotted in Fig. 7 and tabulated in Fig. 8 by vertebrae type.

	C7	T1	T4	T7	T10	L1	L2	L3	L4	L5	S	Lumbar	Overall
Mean error (mm)	5.0	3.4	2.2	3.4	3.3	2.7	3.0	3.2	3.0	2.7	6.5	3.5	3.3
Std in error (mm)	0.0	4.4	1.4	2.8	2.8	2.1	2.4	2.8	2.4	2.1	5.9	3.0	3.2
Mean vert. width (mm)	19.4	19.6	23.9	27.9	32.7	36.0	37.6	38.4	38.8	37.8	31.4	36.6	30.0
Labelled count	1	2	9	25	151	241	249	255	254	254	264	1517	2293
Labelled count (+/- 1)	1	4	13	27	169	271	280	286	284	269	264	1654	2532
Total count	7	11	20	33	181	291	291	291	291	291	291	1746	2726
Labelling rate	14%	18%	45%	76%	83%	83%	86%	88%	87%	87%	91%	86.9%	84.1%
Labelling rate (+/- 1)	14%	36%	65%	82%	93%	93%	96%	98%	98%	92%	91%	94.7%	92.9%

Fig. 8 Localization errors. The mean and standard deviation (std) of localization errors are shown for all the correctly detected and labelled vertebrae (identication rate 84 % overall and 87 % for lumbar). In adittion the "count"—the number of vertebrae detected of each type—is provided, along with the mean width of each of the vertebrae in training set. By allowing the labelling to be correct to +/−1 vertebrae, the identication rates become 93 and 95 % for all and lumbar vertebrae respectively

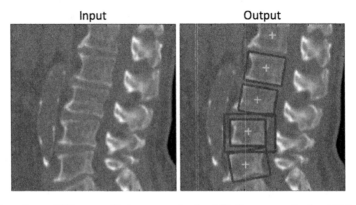

Fig. 9 Detection on CT images with detectors trained on MR. Detectors trained on MR images can also successfully localize vertebrae in CT scans, indicating the robustness of the method to varying image appearance

We achieve 84.1 % correct identification rate overall, and 86.9 % for the lumbar vertebrae. The mean detection error between the Ground Truth centre of the vertebrae and the center of the detected bounding box is 3.3 mm, with standard deviation 3.2 mm. If the assigned labels are allowed to be shifted by +/− one, the errors are 92.9 and 94.7 % respectively.

Independent sacrum detection (without graphical model) with local non-maxima supression shows 98.1 % recall at 48 % precision. Independent general vertebrae detection (without graphical model) shows 97.1 % recall at 9.1 % precision.

Our method works well on very challenging examples with various anomalies illustrated earlier in Fig. 2. The identification results compare favourably to other approaches in the literature, although direct comparison is not possible since the algorithms have been evaluated on different datasets. Glocker et al. [18] report median identification error of 81 % with median localization error below 6mm on CT images. Zhan et al. [15] detect disks and vertebrae in isotropic MRI scans with 97.7 %

"perfect" labelling rate as assessed by a medic but do not report detection errors. Pekar et al. [19] report 83 % correct labelling rate on 30 lumbar MRI scans. Our method is able to correctly localize the centre of the vertebrae out of the mid-sagittal slice in scoliotic cases such as image f in Fig. 6.

Application to CT images. Although the method has been principally designed for MRI images, it is directly applicable to CT images as shown in Fig. 9. No retraining is required for detection on CT due to the high generalization of HOG detectors.

4 Conclusion

We have presented a HOG-based algorithm to localize vertebrae in lumbar MRI scans of the spine that is simple, accurate and efficient. We demonstrate robustness to severe deformations due to diseases, image artefacts, and a wide range of resolution, patient position, and acquisition protocols on a challenging clinical dataset. It is straightforward to extend the method to completely general FOVs if required, by taking other anatomical context into account [18].

Acknowledgments Acknowledgements for the dataset.

References

1. Felzenszwalb, P., Mcallester, D., Ramanan, D.: A discriminatively trained, multiscale, deformable part model. In: Proceedings of CVPR (2008)
2. Pfirmann, C.W.A., Metzdorf, A., Zanetti, M., Hodler, J., Boos, N.: Magnetic resonance classification of lumbar intervertebral disc degeneration. Spine **26**(17), 1873–1878 (2001)
3. Fardon, D.F., Milette, P.C.: Nomenclature and classification of lumbar disc pathology. Spine **26**(5), E93–E113 (2001)
4. Alomari, R.S., Corso, J.J., Chaudhary, V., Dhillon, G.: Desiccation diagnosis in lumbar discs from clinical mri with a probabilistic model. In: IEEE International Symposium on Biomedical Imaging: From Nano to Macro. ISBI '09, pp. 546–549 (2009)
5. Alomari, R.S., Corso, J.J., Chaudhary, V., Dhillon, G.: Computer-aided diagnosis of lumbar disc pathology from clinical lower spine MRI. Int. J. Comput. Assist. Radiol. Surg. **5**(3), 287–293 (2010)
6. Ghosh, S., Alomari, R.S., Chaudhary, V., Dhillon, G.: Computer-aided diagnosis for lumbar mri using heterogeneous classifiers. In: IEEE International Symposium on Biomedical Imaging: From Nano to Macro (2011)
7. Michopoulou, S., Costaridou, L., Vlychou, M., Speller, R., Todd-Pokropek, A.: Texture-based quantification of lumbar intervertebral disc degeneration from conventional t2-weighted MRI. Acta Radiol. **52**(1), 91–98 (2011)
8. Ghosh, S., Alomari, R.S., Chaudhary, V., Dhillon, G.: Automatic lumbar vertebra segmentation from clinical ct for wedge compression fracture diagnosis. In: SPIE 7963, Medical Imaging 2011: Computer-Aided Diagnosis (2011)
9. Wels, M., Kelm, B.M., Tsymbal, A., Hammon, M., Soza, G., Sühling, M., Cavallaro, A., Comaniciu, D.: Multi-stage osteolytic spinal bone lesion detection from ct data with internal

sensitivity control. In: Proceedings of SPIE 8315, Medical Imaging 2012: Computer-Aided Diagnosis (2012)

10. Dalal, N., Triggs, B.: Histogram of oriented gradients for human detection. In: Proceedings of CVPR, vol. 2, pp. 886–893 (2005)

11. Fischler, M., Elschlager, R.: The representation and matching of pictorial structures. IEEE Trans. Comput. **c–22**(1), 67–92 (1973)

12. Felzenszwalb, P., Huttenlocher, D.: Pictorial structures for object recognition. IJCV **61**(1), 55–79 (2005)

13. Oktay, A.B., Akgul, Y.S.: Simultaneous localization of lumbar vertebrae and intervertebral discs with SVM based MRF. IEEE Trans. Med. Imaging 1179–1182 (2013)

14. Ghosh, S., Malgireddy, M.R., Chaudhary, V., Dhillon, G.: A new approach to automatic disc localization in clinical lumbar MRI: Combining machine learning with heuristics. In: International Symposium on Biomedical Imaging (2012)

15. Zhan, Y., Maneesh, D., Harder, M., Zhou, X.S.: Robust MR spine detection using hierarchical learning and local articulated model. Med. Image Comput. Comput.-Assist. Interv.—MICCAI—LNCS **7510**, 141–148 (2012)

16. Chwialkowski, M.P., Shile, P.E., Pfeifer, D., Parkey, R.W., Peshock, R.M.: Automated localization and identification of lower spinal anatomy in magnetic resonance images. Comput. Biomed. Res. **24**(2) (1989)

17. Aslan, M.S., Ali, A., Rara, H., Farag, A.A.: An automated vertebra identification and segmentation in CT images. In: Proceedings of IEEE 17th International Conference on Image Processing (2010)

18. Glocker, B., Feulner, J., Criminisi, A., Haynor, D.R., Konukoglu, E.: Automatic localization and identification of vertebrae in arbitrary field-of-view ct scans. In: Medical Image Computing and Computer-Assisted Intervention (2012)

19. Pekar, V., Bystrov, D., Heese, H.S., Dries, S.P.M., Schmidt, S., Grewer, R., Harder, C.J.D., Bergmans, R.C., Simonetti, A.W., Muiswinkel, A.M.V.: Automated planning of scan geometries in spine mri scans. In: Medical Image Computing and Computer-Assisted Intervention, vol. 10, pp. 601–608 (2007)

20. Alomari, R.S., Corso, J.J., Chaudhary, V.: Labeling of lumbar discs using both pixel- and object-level features with a two-level probabilistic model. IEEE Trans. Med. Imaging **30**(1), 1–10 (2011)

21. Kelm, B.M., Wels, M., Zhou, K.S., Seifert, S., Suehling, M., Zheng, Y., Comaniciu, D.: Spine detection in ct and mr using iterated marginal space learning. Med. Image Anal (2012)

22. Klinder, T., Ostermann, J., Ehm, M., Franz, A., Kneser, R., Lorenz, C.: Automated model-based vertebra detection, identification, and segmentation in CT images. Med. Image Anal. **13**(3), 471–482 (2009)

23. Felzenszwalb, P.F., Grishick, R.B., McAllester, D., Ramanan, D.: Object detection with discriminatively trained part based models. IEEE PAMI **32**(9), 1627–1645 (2010)

24. Potesil, V., Lootus, M., El-Labban, A., Kadir, T.: Landmark localization in images with variable field of view. In: International Symposium on Biomedical Imaging (2013)

Printed in the United States
By Bookmasters